Would You

- How to halt or reverse the aging processes and stay younger longer?
- Which specific foods can prolong your life?
- How to prevent cancer, arthritis, heart disease, and other killer diseases?
- Which special vitamins and certain drugs can prevent premature aging and help you to live a long and healthy life?
- How some popular "life-extension" fads can actually shorten your life?
- The real truth about Gerovital, cell-therapy, and hormone replacement therapy?
- How to protect yourself from youth-destroying and lifeshortening effects of X-rays, free-radicals, cross-linkage, and environmental poisons?
- Why sexual virility and long life go hand in hand, and what you can do to enhance it?
- How to prevent wrinkles, and other visible signs of aging, and look young and beautiful at any age?

If you would like to know the answers to these questions and learn about the latest scientific discoveries, treatments, and techniques which can slow, halt, or reverse the aging processes —

READ THIS BOOK

by an internationally recognized authority on longevity and the world's leading expert on nutrition and holistic medicine.

IT MAY BE A TURNING POINT IN YOUR HEALTH AND YOUR LIFE!

Worldwide Secrets for

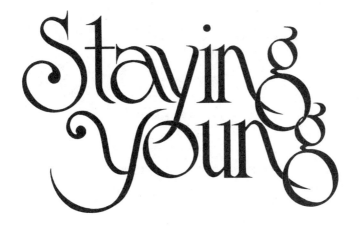

Staying Young

Proven and effective ways to halt and reverse the aging processes and live a long and healthy life—by a world-famous authority

Dr. Paavo Airola

America's foremost nutritionist and leading authority on holistic medicine.
Author of international best-sellers *How To Get Well*, *Are You Confused?*, and *Everywoman's Book*.

HEALTH PLUS, Publishers
P.O. Box 22001, Phoenix, Arizona 85028

WORLDWIDE SECRETS FOR STAYING YOUNG
Copyright © 1982 by
Health Plus Publishers

First Printing, Jan., 1974
Second Printing, Nov., 1975
Third Printing, Dec., 1977
Fourth Printing, May, 1980
Fifth Printing, June, 1981
Sixth, completely revised and updated printing, May, 1982

Publisher's Notes:

1. This book is based on material which originally appeared in a book by the same author, titled *Rejuvenation Secrets From Around The World — That "Work."* It has been completely revised, re-written, and updated. It also contains several new chapters of additional up-to-date information.

2. The information in this book is a compilation of existing data and research by the author. It is offered for educational and research purposes only. The readers should in no way consider the information or directions stated in this book as a substitute for consultation with a duly licensed physician.

Cover photograph of Dr. Airola by Diane Padys, 1979
Typography by Citigraphics, Scottsdale, Arizona

ISBN #0-932090-12-5

Printed in the United States of America

TABLE OF CONTENTS

DEDICATION

To my wife, Marsha —

who has contributed to my growth and true happiness — not by teaching, but by being a living example;

whose loving, unselfish, and compassionate nature has helped me to keep my priorities right in this harsh, materialistic world with its relentless pursuits of conspicuous success and power;

who, with understanding and love, has comforted me in times of distress, shared my joys in times of triumph, helped me to realize my true mission in this life, and inspired me to help others by sharing my knowledge with them;

whose magnanimous heart and childlike faith and perception of deep spiritual insights has re-established with conviction this ultimate truism in my consciousness: That we receive only in the measure that we are willing to give; and

whose contagious enthusiasm, youthful exuberance, and joyful spirit are helping me, as I approach the eighth decade of my life, to stay young —

I dedicate this book.

Paavo Airola

LIVING LONG AND STAYING YOUNG:

Unattainable Dream or Scientific Probability?

We are living in the most exciting era of man's history. Headlines with world-shattering events are an everyday occurrence. Age-old traditions are broken and discarded, and totally new values are formed. The pace of living is accelerated to an unprecedented tempo. Man's relations, not only to his fellow man, but also to his total environment, are undergoing dramatic changes. When the final history of mankind is written, the 20th century will be known by many descriptive labels. My humble contribution to the long list of fitting epithets includes:

- "The Century of Misguided Scientific Progress . . ."
- "The Slow-Extinction-Through-Chemistry Era . . ."
- "The Age of Unholy Alliance Between Science and Food-Drug-Chemical Industries."

But, perhaps, the most appropriate epithet of all for the second half of the twentieth century would be:

- "The Adulation-of-Youth Era."

Modern men and women are searching unrelentingly for ways and means to prolong youth and prevent the aging processes. Interest in methods of preventing premature aging and staying younger longer has never been as keen as it is at the present time. Hundreds of books are written on this subject. No-aging diets, youth-drugs, hormone-treatments, wraps, gadgets, face lifts, face peels, masks, herbs, cellular injections, cosmetic surgery, etc., are developed to fill the growing demand for the preservation and restoration of youth, or extension of life. Plastic surgeons and "youth doctors" make fortunes on the "adulation-of-youth" fad. We are going to great lengths in our efforts to prevent aging, and not only to *feel*, but also to *look*, younger.

Even our modern science is engaged in a search for ways to prolong man's life and prevent the diseases and symptoms of aging. A special branch of medical science, gerontology, is busy working in research centers around the world to solve the secrets of aging and find ways to prolong life. Some startling discoveries have been made in various parts of the world, but especially in Russia, Japan, Germany, and the United States. I will share with you in this book some of these discoveries in the art of staying young and living long.

Age-old Quest.

The search for the secrets of eternal youth — slowing the inevitable aging processes, living a long life, and prolonging health and youthful vitality — is not a phenomenon peculiar to the present day. Man has sought the Fountain of Youth since the dawn of history. Records from early medical history show that a variety of herbs and foods were used to retard the aging processes and revitalize aging bodies. Papyrus of Eber, the oldest medical document known; Chinese records of the Third century; the Hindu doctor Sustrata, 1400 B.C. — all recorded a remarkable interest in the art and science of life-prolongation and prescribed a variety of rejuvenative tonics, herbs, and treatments. The Sumerian King, Gilgamesh, fearing the inevitable decline of life and approaching death, sought desperately the secret herb of eternal life. Legend has it that he finally succeeded in finding the herb, only to have it eaten by a serpent while he was asleep. Most readers are probably familiar with the aging 16th century conquistador, Ponce de Leon, who searched without success for the Fountain of Youth in the New World, and died before reaching threescore and ten.

In the end of the 19th century and in the beginning of the 20th century, some doctors and scientists sought to solve the aging enigma through new medical and scientific insights. Armed with new awareness of the human endocrine system, they began to view the endocrine glands and their secretions, hormones, as possible keys to rejuvenation and life-extension. One of the best-remembered rejuvenation experts is physiologist Charles Edouard Brown-Sequard, who, at the age of 72, tried to rejuvenate himself with injections of dog-testicle extract. Although he claimed that he was remarkably revitalized and felt thirty years younger — he even took a very young wife — he, nevertheless, died a few years later.

Shortly after Brown-Sequard, another European scientist, Dr. Serge Voronoff, attracted the attention — and the monies — of the wealthy by promising rejuvenation in the form of testicular grafts from young monkeys. After making several million dollars from his operations, this original "Youth Doctor" fell into disgrace when it was found that his grafts failed to take, and that he had transferred syphillis from his monkeys to his youth-seeking clients.

More recently, the late Swiss surgeon, Paul Niehans, following in the footsteps of Brown-Sequard and Voronoff, developed so-called cell-therapy. He injected fresh cells from the organs of a sheep fetus into aging bodies and claimed that somehow — he couldn't explain how — the corresponding organs in the human bodies were rejuvenated. Although his famous clinic in Switzerland is still in operation, with thousands of patients treated there every year, many gerontology experts look upon cell-therapy as one of the great rejuvenation frauds of the century.

The Current Life-Extension Frauds and Fakes

Today, in the 80's, the youth cult is at its zenith, especially in the United States. Human history has never known such an incredible interest in rejuvenation and prolongation of life. Why? Perhaps it's our state of general disorientation and confusion. We have discarded the traditional values based on religious ethics, but have failed to establish new values that would give us a sense of orientation and stability. We are haunted by the brevity of earthly existence because our materialistic, de-spiritu-alized, scientifically-oriented thinking cannot accept the traditional beliefs of immortality and eternal life after death. Those who believe in the finality of life at physical death have an obvious desire to prolong this life as much as possible. Those who do not believe in immortality and life everlasting fall easy prey for "life-extension specialists" who promise a few additional years of life on this earth.

Consequently, in youth-oriented America today, there is a virtual avalanche of rejuvenation and life-extension treatments and drugs. So many youth-seekers are search-ing for the ways and means to slow down, halt, and even reverse the aging processes and preserve youth, that we now have new kinds of doctors, clinics, and drugs to supply this fast-growing demand — Youth Doctors, Re-juvenation Clinics, and Life-Extension Drugs. Unfortu-nately, it is becoming more and more apparent that this new field of quasi-medicine, using the respectable name of Gerontology as a cover-up, has been so corrupted and filled with charlatans and quacks, that gullible youth-seekers are being duped, exploited, and relieved of large sums of money in return for which they not only receive worthless rejuvenation treatments, drugs, and injections, but are also risking their health, and even their lives. Although the scientifically and empirically proven, 100% effective, and totally safe ways to prevent premature aging and extend life in optimal health and youthful vitality do exist — as we will see in the following chapters of this book — the Youth Doctors and Life-Extension Specialists do not exhibit much interest in them. Why? Because the true secrets of staying young and living long are linked to our ways of living and eating, to our mental and spiritual attitudes, our state of mind — and you cannot make any money by telling *that* to the youth-seekers! The money is in selling over-priced drugs, injections, gadgets, and mysterious treatments! That's why our life-extension researchers have been directing all their efforts toward finding and developing new drugs that would have a miraculous rejuvenative and life-prolonging effect. Instant youth in a pill! The sad truth is that not only youth-peddling entrepreneurs, but also the youth-seekers themselves prefer such a pill approach. It's much easier to take a pill than to change your lifestyle, develop new eating habits, and adopt a new set of attitudes and values!

Because the American youth-seeking public is now subjected to a fast-growing number of potentially harmful rejuvenative treatments and life-extension drugs, I feel obligated to warn the reader against the use of the following currently-popular materials and fads.

BHT and BHA

BHT (butylated hydroxytolnene) and BHA (butylated hydroxyanisole) are chemical antioxidants used extensively as preservatives in most commercially processed fat-containing foods. The current fad among "longevists" (as some life-extension faddists call themselves) is to take these synthetic man-made preservatives as daily food supplements. They claim that taking these antioxidants orally on a continuous basis will prevent the peroxidation (rancidity) of fats in the body, and, thus, prevent the development of free-radicals, as well as deactivate the existing free-radicals. The medical consensus today is that free-radicals (distorted molecules usually caused by rancidity, radiation, environmental chemicals, stress, etc.) are causatively linked to the development of cancer and other degenerative conditions, as well as premature aging. Preventing the development of free-radicals or deactivating the free-radicals which are already formed in the body would constitute a very important step in preventing the development of the degenerative conditions as well as extending life. But BHT and BHA are dangerous ways to attempt to accomplish this. (I will discuss later in the book how prevention and deactivation of free-radicals can be accomplished by totally natural and harmless means.) There is mounting evidence that BHT and BHA are not completely harmless drugs as some "longevists" claim. There have been reports of undesirable changes in the liver and damage to kidneys and thyroid glands of laboratory animals given these drugs. Loyola University studies show that pregnant mice receiving BHT and BHA produced offspring with abnormal brain chemistry and abnormal behavioral patterns. We don't know enough about the long-term effects of these powerful drugs to recommend them at this time. However, on the basis of what we already do know from a few studies that do exist, BHT and BHA should have no place in any sensible and prudent rejuvenation and life-extension program.

Ethoxyquin, Thiodipropionic Acid, and Nordihydroguaiaretic Acid

These are all synthetic antioxidants which are often used orally by fanatic "longevists." Needless to say, there are no studies that show their usefulness *in humans* as possible free-radical deactivators; nor are there any studies that prove *their harmlessness on a long-term basis.*

RNA and DNA Supplements

Nucleic acids are important dietary factors, but they are so plentiful in a health-oriented nutritionally adequate diet, especially in the Optimum Diet outlined in Chapter 14, that taking them in supplemental form is totally unnecessary. Furthermore, an excess of nucleic acids, especially if taken in an isolated, concentrated form, can be extremely harmful and can severely endanger the health. Nucleic acids metabolize into purines, which in turn form uric acid. There have been many cases of uric acid poisoning and kidney damage, even total kidney failure, caused by excess uric acid, among those who consume large amounts of nucleic-acid-rich foods and/or nucleic acid supplements.

Cell-therapy

Although cell-therapy in various forms is still used in several rejuvenation centers around the world, it is not sanctioned by the medical establishment. There is no scientific evidence that it works; nor how it works, if it does. Since foreign cells are usually rejected by the host's immunological system, it may be that the only possible positive and beneficial action of cell-therapy is due to its stimulating effect on the body's immunological mechanism. An expensive and bothersome way to accomplish that! There are much simpler and easier ways to stimulate the body's immune system, as I will show later in this book.

Hormone-Replacement Treatments

Life-extension scientists have long suspected that the endocrine glands may hold the secret of youth. It is well known that the glandular activity slows down as we age, and the hormone output dwindles. This is particularly true in regard to sex hormones. It is also known that the body loses its ability to make full use of its own hormones as it ages. Scientists—always on the look-out for the Fountain of Youth in the form of a little white pill— postulated that if the missing or undersupplied hormones could be substituted for by a pill or injection, they would be able to prevent the aging processes and extend human life. Of course, they would have to also administer another hormone or drug that would restore the aging body's ability to properly utilize the injected hormones.

Thus, one of the most popular rejuvenation treatments—hormone-replacement therapy—was born. Postmenopausal women are given estrogen injections. Post-andropausal* men are given testosterone shots. Rejuvenation or life-extension-minded men and women are injected with other hormones as well: aldosterone, vasopressin, corticosteroids, hydrocortisone, pituitary hormones, progesterone, estradiol benzoate, etc. What the hormone treatment proponents overlooked is that the endocrine gland system, which naturally manufactures the hormones, is extremely complex. Each gland influences all the other glands in the system, and the desired effect of any one hormone in the body is dependent on the proper proportions of all the other hormones present. Thus,

---

*) Andropause = male climacteric, similar to female menopause.

administering any one isolated hormone will totally disrupt the whole hormonal system, and may actually do more harm than good. Also, although endocrinologists and "longevists" love to play the role of super-detectives, pointing out all the actions, reactions, functions, and interrelationships of various hormones, enzymes, neurotransmitters, etc., the truth is that no one actually knows (and, my hunch is, never will know) all the details and minute intricate human hormonal, neural, and enzymatic systems. Consequently, all attempts to outsmart and outguess nature by trying to balance, normalize, or enhance its hormonal and enzymatic levels with shots and pills is doomed to fail. So far, every hormone-replacement therapy—*every one of them* — has been a disappointment. Severe side effects have been observed, including the growth of malignant tumors. Furthermore, any claimed benefits have been only of short duration. Consequently, there is no valid evidence that hormone-replacement therapy can prevent aging processes or extend life.

Rejuvenation Secrets That "Work"

The basic message of this book is that although misdirected life-extension scientists, looking for secrets of perpetual youth and long life in the wrong areas, will never find them, *effective, proven, and safe ways to prevent and even reverse the aging processes and extend life do exist.* I will reveal them to you in the following chapters. They are as effective as they are simple — and this last word, perhaps, explains why the scientifically-minded longevity researchers, always anticipating involved and complex solutions to their problems, have not found them. The true secrets of staying young and living long are based on simple common sense. They are totally safe and harmless. They are easy to incorporate into your personalized stay-younger-longer program. Best of all, they are not based on speculation, postulations, or theories, but are already 100% proven empirically and confirmed scientifically.

In my travels and studies in many countries around the world, I have found that natives have used for thousands of years certain herbs or natural foods and food substances to attain their good health and long life. For example, the people of Hunza attribute their exceptional health, youthful vitality and extended longevity to drinking their naturally hard (heavily mineralized) water. Thousands of years of actual application has demonstrated to the natives of Hunza that natural minerals in their water are helping to keep them in excellent health and to give them a long life. Recent scientific studies have shown that natural minerals in drinking water do have a decisive effect on man's health, and can help to prevent many degenerative, life-shortening diseases, such as heart disease, diabetes, and osteoporosis.

In Russia, scientists have discovered that the diet of almost all of their centenarians is rich in natural, raw, unprocessed honey, which is heavily "contaminated" by bee pollen.

In Finland, natives consider their hot saunas absolutely necessary to enjoy good health, prevent disease, and prolong life. Modern science has confirmed that hyperthermia, or periodic artificially-induced fever, the kind the sauna bath creates, has a very beneficial effect on general metabolic processes, and it helps to fight many diseases, including arthritis and cancer—and, thus, prolong life.

In Mexico, scientists have discovered that a certain commonly used herb contains natural male and female sex hormones that can prevent senility and aging processes due to diminished hormone production, which is common with approaching old age.

In Sweden, natives have been using a certain wild fruit which, they claim, gives them a youthful appearance, exceptional health, and a long life. Scientists have found that this native fruit contains huge quantities of vitamin C, which is not only one of the most important substances for optimal health and prevention of disease, but also a powerful natural antioxidant, which combats and destroys free-radicals in the body. Free-radicals are known to cause cancer and are also, perhaps more than anything else, responsible for premature aging and early senility.

Let's, therefore, examine these secrets of staying young and living long, secrets which I have uncovered in my worldwide travels and research, and which now have been both empirically and scientifically proven to be effective in preventing premature aging and extending life.

Please join me in an exciting journey from country to country in search of the True Fountain of Youth!

1

Health and Longevity Secrets from

SWEDEN

Swedish women have long been known for their exceptional beauty, well-proportioned bodies, and luscious complexions, which they enjoy into advanced age. Sweden, a little Scandinavian country, has produced more internationally known beauties for the glamorous world of entertainment, and the Swedish girls have won more Miss World and Miss Universe titles than any other nation. Likewise, Swedish men are tall, handsome, and athletic. Sweden has one of the best health records in the world— the lowest infant mortality rate, and the highest life expectancy of any nation. This, in spite of the fact that Sweden has one of the most rugged and unfriendly climates in the world, with large parts of it being located above the Polar Circle.

I spent many years living in Sweden, and made extensive studies of the Swedish mode of living and their nutritional habits. I came to the conclusion that the exceptional health and beauty of the Swedish people are not unrelated phenomena, but are closely tied to certain elements in their daily diet.

ROSE HIPS — SWEDISH HEALTH AND LONGEVITY SECRET NUMBER ONE!

The health and longevity properties of vitamin C have been recently confirmed by many scientific studies in Russia and the United States. Rose hips are the richest natural source of vitamin C, with the possible exception of acerola cherries. Russians call them "vitamin roses." Rose hips contain twenty to forty times more vitamin C than oranges! They are also rich in bioflavonoids, or vitamin P, and many other vitamins and minerals. Here's how rose hips compare with oranges:

- They have 28% more calcium.
- They have 25% more iron.
- They have 25 *times* more vitamin A!
- They have 20-40 times (depending on the variety) more vitamin C.

Rose hips have been introduced to the health-conscious world relatively recently—as a popular health food fad. But in Sweden, rose hips have been used very extensively for centuries! In fact, rose hips have always formed an essential part of the traditional Swedish diet. Swedes make nutritious soups, delicious vitamin-rich teas, jellies, and desserts from them. In Sweden, rose hips positively do not have the aura of a fad food about them. *All* Swedes use rose hips. They are sold in various forms in *all* food stores—not only health food stores—and are a staple food in the humble cottage as well as in the King's castle.

Because of the generous use of rose hips, the traditional Swedish diet has always been extremely rich in high quality natural vitamin C. Long before vitamin C was discovered, the Swedes, guided by natural instinct, gorged on rose hips, thus saturating their diet with vitamin C, *the health and longevity vitamin number one.*

Rose hips grow wild in Sweden, especially in the northern parts of the country, where there are wide areas covered with bushes from which "hips" are picked in the fall. For the benefit of those who may not know, rose hips are the small (about the size of a cherry), fully ripened orange-red fruits just below the rose flower. Only certain varieties of rose hips are suitable for eating. The best fruit-bearing varieties of roses with the richest content of vitamin C are: Rosa Villosa, Rosa Canina, and Rosa Rugosa.

Collagen — Key to Perpetual Youth

Why are rose hips so important for health and long life?

The latest scientific discoveries (by Drs. J. W. McCormick, Johan Bjorksten, I. Stone, Linus Pauling, Roger Williams, and others) have shown that the aging processes and the degenerative changes of the skin—wrinkles, flabbiness, discoloration, etc.—are caused by physiological changes in collagen, the intercellular cement, which holds all the cells and tissues of the body together. Deterioration is caused primarily by a deficiency of vitamin C in the tissues. Sufficient vitamin C in the diet will keep collagen and other connective tissues strong and elastic, which will result in tight skin and a smooth and lovely complexion.

Collagen is responsible for the stability and tensile strength of practically all the tissues of the body, including the skin, the muscles, and the tissues of all organs and glands. The deficiency of vitamin C brings about the breakdown of this intercellular cement, and as a result of this, the instability and fragility of tissues. A vitamin C deficiency, in addition to adversely affecting your health in many other ways, will make your skin loose and flabby, saggy and lifeless, because of a loss of tension and elasticity. Wrinkles will appear early in life, eyes will lose their lustre, lips their fullness.

There are, of course, many other factors involved in feeding and maintaining a healthy skin, as we will see later in the book. Vitamins A and B-complex, minerals, and essential fatty acids are all important. But the breakdown of collagen, caused by a deficiency of vitamin C, is the main cause of the deterioration processes of the skin, and the primary contributing cause of premature aging.

When you finish reading this book, you will understand that the *secret of staying young is basically the secret of staying healthy*, and vitamin C plays a leading role in helping you to stay healthy, prevent disease, and extend your life in youthful vitality.

How Vitamin C Can Keep You Young

Russian scientists have discovered that vitamin C has a profoundly stimulating effect on the adrenal glands. The adrenal glands secrete over 20 steroid hormones, which are directly involved in keeping your vital bodily processes in a condition of high efficiency. It is generally agreed that a decrease in the output of endocrine hormones—which usually begins in late middle life—is responsible for the symptoms of aging. Russian scientists have demonstrated that substantial daily doses of vitamin C have a rejuvenative, stimulating effect on the glandular activity, and the endocrine hormones are once again produced in the higher levels, similar to those found in younger people. Vitamin C also improves the body's ability to effectively utilize these hormones. It is known that this ability diminishes with age.

The world-famous Nobel Prize Winner, Dr. Linus Pauling, reported that large doses of vitamin C may be effective in increasing male virility. It is a commonly known fact that both fertility and virility have been steadily declining during the last few decades, particularly in the United States. It is also a well-known fact that we have a grand scale vitamin C deficiency in the United States. The U.S. Department of Agriculture reports that 48% of all Americans have diets deficient in vital nutritive elements. Vitamin C was found to be one of the substances most lacking in the American diet. "Of the thousands of chemical tests on human adults to determine the body level of vitamin C, 90% were found deficient," said one of the world's leading vitamin C authorities, Dr. J. W. McCormick.

The healthy function of sex glands is directly related to the general health, and to the prolonged feeling and appearance of youth. The first signs of aging usually appear when sex hormone production begins to slow down. A Japanese doctor, M. Higuchi, has demonstrated that there is a relationship between vitamin C levels and the hormone production of the sex glands —the more vitamin C in the diet, the more sex hormones are produced by the glands. Prostatic fluid, which nourishes the sperm and keeps them alive, is extremely rich in vitamin C. A prolonged deficiency in vitamin C can slow down the hormone production of the sex glands and consequently contribute to premature aging.

Furthermore, there is a growing body of evidence that the aging process is largely a matter of the diminished oxygenation of cells. Vitamin C has a great effect on improved cell breathing, and, thus, can help prevent premature aging.

Hardening of the arteries, atherosclerosis, and heart attacks are true diseases of premature aging. Many doctors believe that "you are as old as your arteries." Boris Sokoloff, M.D., Director of the Southern Bio-Research Institute in Florida, reported that their conclusions, based on research and wide-spread evidence from medical literature, is that ascorbic acid (vitamin C) is the key factor in averting atherosclerosis, and, thus, preventing heart disease, our number one killer.

German professor, Werner Grab, M.D., has stated that vitamin C not only has curative powers in such diseases as hepatitis, influenza, rheumatic diseases, polio, metabolic diseases, and acute poisonings, but that even cancer will be inhibited by huge doses of ascorbic acid.

Vitamin C: Natural Antioxidant and Free-radical Deactivator

Several current studies, particularly those by Drs. Cameron and Pauling, show that vitamin C can also have a curative effect on cancer, even in advanced stages. According to reports of famous researchers, Drs. Raymond Schamberger and Nicolas Petrakis, one of the prime causes of many cancers, especially cancers of the breast and colon, is so-called free-radicals. Free-radicals are the result of lipid peroxidation. Lipids (oils and fats) combine with oxygen to form peroxides, aldehydes, and malonaldehydes. These damaged fat molecules turn into harmful free-radicals. Free-radicals not only cause cancer and contribute to several other degenerative conditions, they also cause cross-linkage in fibrous protein tissues of the body—collagen, elastin, and reticulin of the connective tissues. Cross-linkage changes the usually pliable, elastic, and resilient collagen tissue into a tough and less resilient tissue. The skin becomes wrinkled and leathery. The joints and cartilage become stiff and less mobile. Arteries lose their rubbery ability to freely expand and contract, and become hardened. All this gradually impairs many of the essential body processes. Vital organs and glands cannot function properly, the general health gradually deteriorates, and the aging processes set in.

But, hear this: Vitamin C is one of the most effective natural antioxidants and free-radical deactivators! It prevents lipid peroxidation and formation of free-radicals in the body. Not only this, but even when the health has already deteriorated considerably and there is substantial free-radical formation, vitamin C can deactivate existing free-radicals and prevent the destruction of collagen by cross-linkage.

As you can see, vitamin C is, indeed, a very important factor in preventing premature aging and staying younger longer.

Vitamin C also has many other vital functions in the body that add to the total balance of extending your youthfulness to an advanced age. It is essential for effective assimilation of iron, calcium, and other minerals. It helps to regulate cholesterol levels. It is used for the formation of many enzymes and hormones. It increases the body's resistance to infections; it helps to destroy dangerous pathogenic bacteria and viruses. It is also a great detoxifier. It neutralizes and/or destroys most of the toxins (endogenous and exogenous) in the body and helps to excrete them from the system. In this age of universal pollution, this is extremely important. Vitamin C can protect you against the toxicity of lead, mercury, cadmium, aluminum, benzene, and many other environmental and industrial chemical pollutants. In addition, vitamin C can help protect you from, or cure, many of the diseases that orthodox medicine is totally helpless against, such as herpes, flu, the common cold, arthritis, and mononucleosis.

Vitamin C—The True Fountain of Youth!

As you can see, if there ever has been a true miracle rejuvenative substance, vitamin C is it. It has so many universal applications that it is virtually impossible to find a condition of ill health or diminished well-being which vitamin C would not affect favorably, very often with a miraculous healing effect. Since old age is often associated with various conditions of diminished health, it stands to reason that vitamin C should be rejuvenative tonic number one for anyone over 40 years of age. Vitamin C is completely non-toxic in doses up to 5,000 mg. a day on a regular basis. A natural form of vitamin C, such as rose hips, is preferable, as it is accompanied by other vitamins of the C-complex, such as hesperidin, rutin, citrin, etc., which are generally called bioflavonoids. Bioflavonoids act as synergists with vitamin C, increasing its effect and making it biologically more potent. But since it is impossible to obtain 100% natural vitamin C from rose hips in large doses, the ascorbic acid, sodium ascorbate, or calcium ascorbate forms of vitamin C can be used. Although 3,000 to 5,000 mg. a day is sufficient for most adults, those who are under extreme emotional or physical stress, recuperating from an illness, or subject to extreme toxic environmental poisons or heavy air pollution, could take up to 10,000 mg. a day.

WHEY — SWEDISH HEALTH AND LONGEVITY SECRET NUMBER TWO

Whey is the liquid leftover of the cheese-making process. When the milk coagulates, the solid part — curds — is removed and the remaining liquid is called whey. In the United States, whey is usually thrown away or sold as a by-product for animal feed.* In Sweden, whey is never wasted; in fact, it is a national food. It is dehydrated and made into whey cheese (mesost) and whey butter (messmör).

In earlier times, when the Swedish dairy was neither industrialized nor mechanized, whey cheese and

---

*) Only recently, after I enthusiastically glamorized the health-giving and rejuvenative properties of whey in one of my earlier books, *Health Secrets From Europe*, did whey appear on the shelves of health food stores as a food supplement.

whey butter were made directly on the farms. Liquid whey was boiled in large iron kettles over the fire until the water evaporated, and the semi-solid whey remained. Then the whey was put into cloth or wooden forms to harden into cheese-like shapes and consistency — whey cheese. It was also put into glass jars and mixed with cream to form a butter-like spread — whey butter. Even now, in some parts of Sweden, Norway, and Finland, whey cheese and whey butter are made on the farms in this manner. However, today the bulk of all whey products in Sweden is made in modern dairy factories by a modern evaporating process.

Colonic Hygiene — Secret of Eternal Youth

Here are some scientific reasons why I consider whey to be an important health and longevity factor in the Swedish diet.

Of all the "secrets" of perpetual youth which man has uncovered and tried in his long search, perhaps none is more scientifically established than one which is based on the premise that *colonic hygiene*—or the perfectly and efficiently functioning digestive, assimilative, and eliminative system—is the real secret of eternal youth.

Ilja Metchnikoff, the eminent Russian bacteriologist, made revolutionary discoveries at the turn of the century in regard to ways of prolonging life. He believed that autotoxemia (self-poisoning) through putrefaction of metabolic wastes in the small and large intestines is the main cause of premature aging.

Your intestines house billions of bacteria which help your digestive system to break down the food you eat, and, thus, aid in the digestion and assimilation of nutrients. Many important nutrients, including some of the B vitamins, are produced in the intestines by these intestinal bacteria. For optimum health, it is extremely important that there is always a plentiful supply of these beneficial bacteria. Metchnikoff discovered that soured milks, and such milk products as whey, help feed the bacteria in the intestines and prevent the development of harmful putrefactive bacteria which lead to autotoxemia. The more beneficial bacteria present in the colon, the less toxins produced by the putrefactive bacteria. Whey, which contains lactose, is the best natural food for these friendly intestinal bacteria.

Thus, whey is perhaps the best food for preventing self-poisoning due to intestinal putrefaction, intestinal sluggishness, and constipation. Whey can also aid in the assimilation of nutrients from the foods you eat.

Constipation—Enemy of Health and Longevity

Many scientists believe that chronic intestinal sluggishness and constipation, together with faulty nutrition and poor digestion and assimilation of food, are the major contributing factors to many, if not most, illnesses and premature aging. The toxins, or poisons created by bacterial metabolism and putrefaction, remain in the intestines, and, as a result of prolonged constipation, are absorbed into the blood and, consequently, poison the whole organism. Thus, constipation can be directly linked to many rheumatic and arthritic conditions, eczema and other skin disorders, bad breath, chronic headaches, nervous conditions, digestive disorders, colitis, and diverticulitis.

Whey is up to 77% lactose, which is a natural food for the friendly acidophilus and bifidus bacteria in the intestines. It has been scientifically established that using whey regularly will prevent constipation, internal sluggishness, gas, and bowel putrefaction.

27

Constipation is a number one enemy of beauty, too. A woman with a serious constipation problem can be spotted instantly; her skin has a muddy, gray tone; it is rough, porous, and often covered with eczema, pimples, and other blemishes; her breath is foul because her abused body is trying to purify its blood through the lungs. This was well understood by Cleopatra, famous for her clear, velvety, unblemished and lusciously fresh complexion. According to Cleopatra's historian, Estelle Erlan, Cleopatra's "beauty secret" was her regular cleansing of the system with the mildly laxative leaves of *senna* to prevent constipation and keep her intestinal tract clean.

Scandinavian women—and men—keep their complexions unblemished, clear, and healthy with whey. By preventing constipation and cultivating beneficial vitamin-producing and disease-fighting bacteria in the intestines, whey also helps the Scandinavian people to enjoy excellent health and a longer life in youthful vitality.

In Sweden, whey is eaten daily by everyone. It is sold in all food stores, and you can find it on the table in every Swedish home in the form of cheese or butter.

In addition to being a miraculous cleanser and promoting the growth of beneficial intestinal bacteria, whey is also an excellent food. It is rich in minerals, particularly iron, and vitamins, especially the age-fighting vitamin B_1. Here are a few nutritional facts about Swedish or Norwegian whey cheese:

- 77% of it is pure lactose — the active factor in its favorable influence on the intestinal tract.
- It has only 3.6% butter fat, as compared to 25%-40% for ordinary cheese.
- It has 6 times more iron than beef, twice as much as beans or eggs, and 50% more than liver!

- It has 10 times more vitamin B_1 than ordinary cheese, twice as much as beef, and 5 times as much as milk.

- It has 7 times as much vitamin B_2 as beef, 20 times as much as milk, and 20 times as much as whole wheat flour.

Next to brewer's yeast, whey is the richest natural source of B_1 and B_2; these B-vitamins are extremely important for preserving a youthful appearance and preventing premature aging.

Unfortunately, whey cheese and whey butter are difficult to obtain in the United States. I have been successful in buying some in better cheese and delicatessen shops. *Whey powder* or *whey tablets*, sold in every health food store in the United States, are excellent substitutes for whey cheese and butter, having roughly the same nutritive and therapeutic value.

Make sure to incorporate whey into your diet, especially if you are prone to intestinal sluggishness, gas, or constipation. One or two tablespoons of whey powder a day, mixed with drinks or foods, is the suggested dose. Remember, whey—the health and longevity secret from Sweden—is not a drug, it is a natural miracle food which can help you to stay younger longer.

Health and Longevity Secrets from

FINLAND

The great ancient physician, Parmenides, said two thousand years ago:

"Give me a chance to create fever, and I will cure any disease."

Two giants of modern medicine in Germany, Professor Werner Zabel, M.D., and Dr. Josef Issels, M.D., say:

"Artificially induced fever has the greatest potential in the treatment of many diseases, including cancer."

Med. Prof. Werner Zabel, M.D., told me the following true story:

Until a few decades ago, the great Pontine swamps, not far from Rome, Italy, presented a constant source of malaria infections. Then, by government action, the swamps were dried out and malaria disappeared. But a remarkably strange observation was made recently. While earlier the whole malaria-infected area was free from cancer, now, a generation later, the population there shows the same incidence rate of cancer as the rest of Italy.

Dr. Zabel says that the mystery of the Pontine swamps has a simple solution: the frequent fever attacks, common in malaria patients, stimulated the body's own defenses so that cancer could not develop. Even when cancer had already developed, the exposure to malaria and the accompanying attacks of high fever had a curative effect.

It has also been reported from Italy that there has never been observed any cases of cancer on the island of Sardinia, where practically everyone is affected by malaria.

Fever—Misunderstood Healing Symptom

Fever has been too long a misunderstood and mistreated symptom. Most medical doctors try to combat and suppress fever. They see fever as a negative pathological condition which must be eliminated as fast as possible. With many modern fever-suppressing drugs, they quickly bring the fever down to "normal."

But things are beginning to change, and modern medical science is discovering (re-discovering) the therapeutic value of fever. Particularly in Europe, many biological clinics now use artificially induced fever to treat many of our most common diseases, including cancer. Famous French virologist and Nobel Prize Winner, Dr. A. Lwoff, made extensive research on the physiology of fever and concluded that:

"High temperature during infection helps combat the growth of virus. Therefore, fever should not be brought down with drugs."

Artificially induced fever, used extensively by ancient doctors, has been revived in modern practice by Maria Schlenz of Germany. The famous Schlenz-bath, which she originated, is now used extensively in many biological clinics in Europe. Artificially raised fever is now the cornerstone in the therapeutic program of most biological and holistic medical clinics in Europe. More and more progressive doctors around the world are beginning to understand the true nature of fever and are applying it for healing and preventing disease.

In the United States, artificially induced fever therapy, hyperthermia, is now used in several progressive medical centers, mostly in the treatment of cancer. Various methods of inducing fever are used: electric wraps, special fever-inducing vaccines and drugs, etc.

How Fever "Works"

Your body is equipped with the most intricate and effective defensive and healing system. When you subject yourself to various stresses of life, or when your body is attacked by hostile organisms, your defensive system initiates various protective measures to meet the demands of stress. A complex glandular system— particularly the lymphatic glands, tonsils, and endocrine glands—forms a defensive line against hostile invaders, poisons, or other stress factors which pose a threat to your health or your life. If this first Maginot Line of defense is broken, your body initiates more drastic measures for correcting the conditions that threaten your health and your life. Fever is one of these defensive and healing measures. The high temperature speeds up metabolism, inhibits the growth of the invading virus or bacteria, and literally burns the enemy with heat. This is not wishful thinking, but a solidly established scientific fact, proven by Dr. A. Lwoff in many experiments. Fever is an effective protective and healing measure, not only against colds, simple infections, and muscular pains, but also such serious ailments as polio, cancer, rheumatic diseases, and skin disorders.

How Finns Use Fever to Stay Healthy and Young

While modern medical science is in the process of re-discovering the therapeutic benefits of fever, Finnish people have been using artificially created fever for centuries. After discovering instinctively the invigorating, health-promoting, and rejuvenating effect of heat on their bodies, Finns have built steam-bath houses—saunas—and have made sauna-bathing a national tradition unparalleled in history. In fact, Finland, this little, cold Northern country with the rugged, honest, and brave people, is known around the world mainly for three reasons: (1) It is the only country that has paid all of its debts to the United States; (2) It is the only country that won its war with Russia (1939-40) and retained independence; and (3) It is the originator of the now famous sauna, the popularity of which is spreading worldwide.

Sauna, the Finnish steambath, is an historic tradition in Finland. For over a thousand years, the sauna has been an important part of Finnish life and Finnish culture — cherished by every Finnish man, woman, and child. The sauna is credited with being a most important reason for the rugged vitality and endurance — the *sisu* —of the Finnish people; also for their exceptional health and low incidence of such degenerative diseases as cancer and arthritis.

In a country of approximately 5 million people, there are an estimated 700,000 steam bath facilities — one sauna for every 7 people! Most Finnish saunas are in buildings specially constructed for this purpose. Every farm has its own sauna, normally built on the shore of a lake or river. Most family dwellings in the city have a sauna built on the lot, usually in the back yard. In most apartment buildings, special sauna rooms are constructed in the basement. All cities and towns have a large number of public saunas where those few Finns who do not have their own private saunas go at least once or twice a week.

The traditional Finnish sauna is a so-called smoke sauna. It is a timber structure, about 12 by 18 feet, divided into two chambers — the dressing room, and the steam room. The dressing room has several benches to rest on while cooling down after the bath. The steam room has a large oven built from field stones, which are heated by a wood fire. There is no chimney — smoke fills the room while the sauna is being heated up. There is a large iron cauldron built into the oven for hot water. A barrel of cold water is also in the bathing room. There is a window, and a ventilation shutter. Stair-type benches of various heights are built on one side of the room. The sauna is ready for use when the rocks in the oven are hot. Then the fire is put out, the room is well ventilated to remove the rest of the smoke, and the sauna is ready. Of course, the more modern types of Finnish saunas are now built so that the smoke does not enter the room at all, although rocks are always used. In some newer models, the rocks are heated by electric heat.

In Finland, the whole family normally takes a bath together. Sometimes, especially in large families with servants and guests, all the men go together first; then all the women have a group bath. The sauna is always taken on Saturday evenings, sometimes also in the middle of the week.

The Finnish sauna starts with *löyly*, which is the Finnish word for steam. Water is thrown over the hot rocks, hot steam fills the room and raises the temperature. The bather can sit on the desired level of the stair-like benches, depending on the temperature he prefers

— the higher the bench, the higher the temperature. The usual temperature for a Finnish sauna is about 200-210° F, sometimes even higher. However, for the uninitiated, I would not advise temperatures higher than 180-190° F.

In order to further increase the effect of heat and to stimulate sweating and raise the body's temperature, the Finns use birch brooms—*vihta*. Fresh birch branches with leaves are tied together in a bundle to form a short broom. They are used fresh in the summer, or dried in the winter. The dried broom is dipped in warm water and it immediately regains the same shape as the fresh one. Bathers hit themselves all over with these birch brooms. It may seem odd and eccentric to the uninitiated, but you have to try it yourself to appreciate the fantastic delight and unbelievable pleasure that sauna with a birch broom can give!

Following the sauna with hot *löyly*, bathers wash themselves with warm water and soap, and then take a long, relaxing rest on the benches in the dressing room, allowing their wide-open pores to close slowly, perspiration to cease, and the body to return slowly to normal temperature.

Since saunas are becoming more and more popular in the United States, and since there is so much misunderstanding and misinformation regarding the correct way to build and use the sauna, I wish to emphasize these two points:

1. The Finnish sauna is never a *dry* sauna. The heat in the authentic Finnish sauna is always created by throwing water over the hot rocks — thus, it is a moist, steam heat.

2. Finns do not end their saunas by cooling themselves rapidly with a cold shower, as is often advised in the United States. Even when Finns, while taking a sauna, swim in the lake or river or roll in the soft snow

during the winter, they always go back to the hot sauna for a second session, and then finish the whole ceremony by taking a long rest on the dressing room benches and letting the body return *slowly* to normal temperature. This is important, as the healing and rejuvenating effects of the sauna are largely due to the raised body temperature, and to cool it down suddenly with a cold shower would be to interrupt a beneficial process and possibly cause harm.

Why Sauna Heals and Rejuvenates

The therapeutic and rejuvenative property of the sauna is attributed to the following facts:

- Overheating with *löyly* stimulates and speeds up the metabolic processes and inhibits the growth of pathogenic bacteria or viruses.
- The vital organs and glands, including endocrine and sex glands, are stimulated to increase activity.
- The body's own healing activity and restorative capacity are accelerated and increased. The healing of many chronic and acute conditions, such as colds, infections, rheumatic diseases, and cancer is accelerated by the body's own curative forces.
- The body is thoroughly cleansed and rejuvenated inside and outside. The sauna brings about profuse sweating. Many toxins, accumulated in the system as a result of metabolic wastes and sluggish elimination, are thrown out of the body with perspiration. The skin is our largest eliminative organ — 30% of all body wastes are normally eliminated by way of perspiration. The chemical analysis of sweat shows that it contains almost the same constituents as urine (skin is appropriately called our "third kidney"). The sauna increases the eliminative, detoxifying, and cleansing capacity of the skin by the stimulating action on the sweat glands.

It is easy to see why Finnish people are known for their rugged health, stamina, and youthful vigor.

How You Can Use Fever for Health and Rejuvenation

If you are fortunate enough to have your own sauna, or have access to one, take a sauna once or twice a week. Follow the Finnish method, and *do not cool yourself with a cold shower immediately after the sauna.* Wrap yourself in a large bath towel to preserve the body heat, and let your body cool down slowly by resting for half an hour or longer.

If you do not have access to a sauna, you can benefit from overheating therapy by taking a Schlenz-bath regularly, or by taking an improvised do-it-yourself sauna in your bed. Here's how you do it.

SCHLENZ-BATH

Fill your bath tub with warm water, about 102° F. If you don't have a large enough tub to enable you to cover your whole body with water, plug the emergency outlet with a piece of cloth or paper so that the water level can be raised (but be careful not to flood your house!). Stay *under* the water as completely as possible, leaving only the face out for breathing. Let hot water run slowly from the faucet so that the temperature of the water is maintained at 102° or 103° F. After about half an hour, your body temperature will match the temperature of the water, if you are totally immersed. Then dry yourself, wrap with a large, dry bath towel, and go to bed, covered with a warm blanket. Stay in bed and continue sweating for as long as possible — maybe an hour or more — until your body temperature gradually returns to normal.

Caution:
1. Do not eat for at least two hours before the bath.
2. Sauna exerts a great stress on the heart and cardiovascular system. Therefore, moderation in temperature and frequency is advisable.
3. Those who suffer from any kind of illness, but particularly high blood pressure and heart disease, should ask their doctor about the advisability of using hot baths, and should abide by his expert advice.

DO-IT-YOURSELF SAUNA

Wrap yourself in a large, heavy bath towel. Put a plastic or rubber sheet on your bed to protect it from damage from perspiration. Take two or three hot water bottles (or electric heating pads) and lay on the rubber sheet. Cover yourself with an electric blanket turned on high, leaving just a crack for breathing. Use several heavy blankets if necessary. Remain until profuse sweating occurs — half an hour or more. Then dry yourself and rest in bed again for awhile until the body is slowly cooled down.

In conclusion, a piece of advice: physical activity to the point of heavy perspiration is almost as beneficial, if not more so, than the overheating bath. Physical exertion may actually raise body temperature several degrees. A combination of regular heavy exercise, such as running, jogging, or active games, resulting in profuse perspiration, can substitute for a Finnish sauna.

FINNISH HEALTH AND LONGEVITY
SECRET NUMBER TWO—RYE

My worldwide studies show that all people known for their excellent health always use some kind of grain as a staple in their diet. In Russia, it is wheat, buckwheat and millet. In Mexico, it is corn and beans. In China and Japan, it is rice. In the Middle East, it is sesame seeds. In East Europe, it is barley and wheat. In Scotland, it is oats. Grains, legumes, seeds, and nuts are the most important and most potent foods for man's health. Their nutritional value is unsurpassed by any other food. Eaten mostly raw (nuts) and sprouted (seeds), but also cooked (grains), they contain all the important nutrients essential for human growth, maintenance of health, and prevention of disease in the most perfect combination and balance. In addition, they contain the secret of life itself—*the germ*—the reproductive power that assures the perpetuation of the species. This reproductive power is of extreme importance for the life of man, his health, and his own reproductive capacity.

All seeds and grains are useful and beneficial, but some grains are more so than others. Millet and buckwheat contain complete proteins of high quality, which most other grains do not contain. Rye, wheat, rice, and corn do not contain all the essential amino acids which form high quality proteins. Furthermore, many vital nutrients in grains, such as minerals, and particularly the trace minerals manganese, iron, copper, molybdenum, and zinc, are not well utilized by the body as they are "locked in" by phytin, which the human digestive system is unable to break down.

Rye has been a staple in the Finnish diet for centuries, mostly in the form of rye bread. But Finns eat mostly *sourdough* rye bread, which is one of the secrets of their exceptional health. According to Dr. Johannes Kuhl (see the next chapter), the famous German expert on soured (lactic acid) foods, the fermentation of grains makes many nutrients more easily available for assimilation in the intestinal tract. During the natural souring process in making sourdough bread, the phytin is broken down and valuable minerals and trace elements are released. Also, during fermentation, due to the enzymatic action on the grain, valuable lactic acid develops—an extremely beneficial health-promoting and disease-preventing factor, as demonstrated by Dr. Kuhl and others in actual studies.

Sourdough rye bread is also extremely beneficial for the health of the digestive and eliminative organs. Being a "predigested" food, it is easily digested and utilized even by weak organs. It is also an *anti-constipation food* — while most other grains are just the opposite! And, as you remember from the previous chapter, chronic constipation is one of the prime causes of most degenerative diseases, as well as of premature aging. Here's how to make

SOURDOUGH RYE BREAD

8 cups freshly ground whole rye flour
3 cups warm water
½ cup sourdough culture

Mix 7 cups of flour with the water and sourdough culture. Cover and let stand in a warm place for 12-18 hours. Add remaining flour, mix well, and knead for 5 minutes, using a dough mixer if you have one. Place in buttered and floured pans. Let rise in a warm place for approximately 1-2 hours, or until the loaf has risen noticeably. Always save ½ cup of dough as a culture for the next baking. Keep the culture in your refrigerator. For the initial baking, it will be necessary to obtain a sourdough culture from a friend or from a commercial baker.

Preheat oven to 350°-400° F. and bake for 1 hour, or more, if needed. This recipe makes one 2-pound loaf. Sourdough bread baking is a delicate art. If you do not succeed at first, don't give up — keep experimenting until you bake a sublimely delicious loaf that will not only fill your house with Old-Country aroma, but will delight your family and justify the Biblical reference to bread as the "Staff of Life."

3

Health and Longevity Secrets from

GERMANY

Germans are, perhaps, more health conscious than any other people I know. They have, for example, the thousands-of-years-long tradition of *bads* — health spas, mineral baths and hot springs, where they go for a *cure*. There are several hundred famous *bads* in Germany, where an estimated three million people go each year to improve their health, cure disease, and/or prevent sickness. The private industries and insurance companies in Germany spent an estimated 20 million dollars setting up so-called health rebuilding centers, where executives and workers are sent periodically to have their health rebuilt, their heart conditions corrected, and where they are instructed to follow a special regimen and diet upon their return home, in order to prevent recurrence.

Germany, where modern medical science was born, also leads the world in regard to the "medical science of the future" — biological medicine. Over 3,000 German medical doctors are members of the Society of Biological Doctors, who do not use drugs, but adhere to the naturopathic methods of natural healing. There are numerous biological clinics and spas in Germany run by these doctors, where millions of people are treated yearly. Many of the most successful biological approaches and methods of treatment have originated in these clinics. I will introduce you to some of these treatments.

FERMENTED FOODS

I don't know if the Germans originated sauerkraut, but it has been an essential part of the German diet for centuries. Germans also use a lot of other fermented foods such as black sourdough bread, soured pickles, and soured or pickled vegetables, such as green and red peppers, beets, carrots, etc.

Fermented foods are used in Germany and many East-European countries not only as a food, but also as a medicine. Miraculous cures of arthritis, scurvy, ulcers, colds, digestive disorders, and even cancer have been attributed to the regular use of fermented foods. People have been eating these foods for centuries without knowing why they had such a curative effect.

Now, German cancer researcher, Dr. Johannes Kuhl, M.D., gives us a scientific explanation as to why fermented foods not only can build health and prevent disease, but also cure disease. "Natural lactic acid and fermentive enzymes, which are produced during the fermentation process, have a beneficial effect on metabolism and a curative effect on disease," says Dr. Kuhl.

Lactic acid destroys harmful bacteria in the intestines and contributes to the better digestion and assimilation of nutrients. Fermented foods can be considered to be predigested foods—very easily digested and assimilated even by persons with weak digestive organs. Fermented foods improve intestinal hygiene and provide proper nourishment for the body's own vitamin production within the intestines. They are also excellent preventative foods against constipation.

You can see now why fermented foods, such as sauerkraut, pickled vegetables, sourdough black bread and soured milks have always been regarded by those who use them regularly as health-building and rejuvenating foods.

Here are a few tips regarding fermented foods:

Do not use commercial sauerkraut or dill pickles from your regular supermarket. They are always prepared with vinegar (not to mention several toxic chemicals and preservatives) and can not be considered to be natural lactic acid foods. In fact, they do not contain natural lactic acid.

Make your own fermented foods. Here are some recipes and instructions for homemade sauerkraut, homemade dill pickles, pickled vegetables and soured milks:

HOMEMADE CULTURED MILK

Use only unpasteurized, raw milk. Place a bottle of milk in a pan filled with warm water, and heat it to about body temperature. Fill a cup or a deep plate, stir in a tablespoon of yogurt or cultured buttermilk, cover with a paper towel (to keep dust off) and keep in a warm place — for example, near the stove, radiator, or wherever there is a constant warm temperature. The milk will coagulate in approximately 24 hours.

Use 1 or 2 spoonfuls of soured milk as a culture for your next batch (use yogurt or commercial buttermilk only as a starting culture for the first batch).

HOMEMADE KEFIR

To make your own kefir, you will need kefir grains. Perhaps you can get some from your friends. If not, you can order kefir grains from R.A.J. Biological Laboratory, 35 Park Ave., Blue Point, Long Island, New York.

The kefir grains will last indefinitely — there is never any need to reorder. Merely follow the instructions which will come with the grains. They multiply rapidly, so please, share them with your friends.

Place 1 tablespoon of kefir grains in a glass of milk. Stir and allow to stand at room temperature overnight. When the milk coagulates, it is ready for use. Strain and save the grains for the next batch. Kefir is a true "elixir of youth," used by centenarians in Bulgaria, Russia, and Caucasus as an essential part of their daily diet.

Freeze-dried kefir culture, sold in health food stores, can also be used in making kefir. It is not re-usable, however.

HOMEMADE YOGURT

Heat one quart of skim milk almost to boiling, then cool to room temperature. Add 2-3 tablespoons of plain yogurt. Stir well. Pour into a wide-mouth thermos bottle, cover, and let stand overnight. In lieu of a thermos bottle, you can use an ordinary glass jar, placing it in a pan of warm water over an electric burner switched on "warm" for 4-5 hours, then switch to "off" and let jar remain in warm water until the milk is solid. If you prefer, you can use a convenient automatic yogurt maker, which can be bought in health food stores.

Use 2-3 spoonfuls of your fresh homemade yogurt as a culture for the next batch.

HOMEMADE SAUERKRAUT

Cut white cabbage heads into narrow strips with a large knife or grater, and place in a wooden barrel or an earthenware pot. A large stainless steel pail or a glass container could possibly be used, but under no circumstances use an aluminum utensil.

When the layer of cabbage is about 4 to 6 inches deep, sprinkle with a few juniper berries, cummin seeds, and/or black currant leaves — use your favorite or whatever you have available. A few strips of carrots, green peppers, and onions can also be used. Add a little sea salt — not more than 2 ounces total for each 25 pounds of cabbage. Continue making layers of grated cabbage and spices until the container is filled. Each layer should be pressed and pounded very hard with your fists or a piece of wood so that there will be no air left and the cabbage will be saturated with its own juice.

When the container is full, cover the cabbage with a clean cheesecloth, place a wooden or slate board over it, and on the top place a clean heavy stone. Let stand for 10 days to 2 weeks — longer if the temperature is below 70° F. Now and then remove the foam and possible mildew from the top, from the stone, and from the container's edges. The cheesecloth, board, and stone should occasionally be removed, washed well with warm water and then cold water, and replaced. When the sauerkraut is ready for use, it can be left in the container, which now should be stored in a cold place, or (preferably) put into glass jars and kept in the refrigerator.

Sauerkraut is best eaten raw — both from the point of taste and for its health-giving value. Drink the sauerkraut juice, too. It is an extremely beneficial and wonderfully nutritious drink.

HOMEMADE PICKLED VEGETABLES

Use the same method as described in the recipe for Sauerkraut to make health-giving lactic acid vegetables. Beets, carrots, green and red peppers, beet tops, and celery are particularly adapted for pickling.

After vegetables are washed and chopped to about 1-1½ inch pieces, pack them tightly into a jar or other suitable container, fill the container with water (which must first be boiled, then cooled to room temperature), add salt and spices, place the board or slate on top to keep vegetables under the water, and cover the container with a cloth. Keep in a warm place, not below 70° F. When pickled vegetables are ready, place them, with juice, in glass jars and store in the refrigerator.

HOMEMADE DILL PICKLES

Use only small, fresh, firm cucumbers. Place them in cold water overnight, then remove and dry well.

Place cucumbers in a wooden barrel or a large earthenware or glass container. Put a few leaves of black currants or cherries, caraway or mustard seeds, and several dill branches in with the cucumbers. If fresh dill is not available, use dry dill weed.

Boil a sufficient amount of salt water, using about 4 ounces of sea salt for 5 quarts of water. Let the water cool down, then pour it over the cucumbers. Cover with a cheesecloth, place a wooden board over it, and on the top a clean heavy stone. There should be enough salt water to cover the board. Keep the container in a warm place for about 1 week, then move to a cooler place. Pickles are ready for eating in about 10 days to 2 weeks. It may take a little longer if the temperature is cold. Every 5 days or so, remove the stone and the covers and wash them well, first in warm water, then in cold water, and replace them. Keep the top of the water clear of foam and mildew. When pickles are ready for eating, they can be placed in glass jars and kept in the refrigerator.

MINERAL WATERS

As I said previously, Germany is famous for its *bads* —mineral bathing and drinking spas—where over three million people go each year to heal and rejuvenate themselves.

The water cure is an old tradition in Germany. Cities have been built around mineral-rich springs. Most mineral spring spas are operated by the city or municipal governments and are directed by licensed medical doctors. In Germany, doctors don't frown on the mineral spas as quackery, as American doctors do. On the contrary, most patients who frequent bathing places for a water cure are sent there by their doctors.

I have visited many *bads* in Germany, and interviewed many doctors who operate them, as well as many patients who take the water cure. All were enthusiastic regarding the benefits of drinking mineral waters and taking mineral baths. High blood pressure, arthritis, female disorders, cardiovascular diseases, skin disorders, nervous disorders, allergies, diseases of old age and senility — this is just a partial list of diseases improved or cured in these water spas.

How Mineral Waters Heal and Rejuvenate

There is a new branch of medical science that many researchers in Germany are probing with an intensified inquiry. It is called *Balnealogy* — the medical science of curing and preventing sickness by bathing.

A doctor in one of the most famous bathing places in Germany, Bad Pyrmont, told me:

"The modern inquiry into balnealogy and the medicinal value of mineral waters is recent and as yet incomplete. But what is already known indicates that mineral waters do indeed have curative powers. And they should, inasmuch as disordered mineral metabolism and biochemical derangement are at the root of many diseases. But what is even more important is the fact that these waters here in Bad Pyrmont have been used for healing purposes for almost two thousand years; and millions of sick people have benefited from them — patients and doctors see examples of it every day!"

For many years, it was believed that our bodies can only use *organic* minerals, and that *inorganic* minerals, such as those present in mineral waters, can not be utilized by the body, and can even be harmful. Now, scientists have reversed their opinions completely. Several studies from around the world show that actually inorganic minerals are not only well utilized, but that they are of extreme importance in the maintenance of health.

Drs. Korenyi, Harkavy, and Whittier reported on the experiments they conducted with 35 patients with high cholesterol levels at the Creedmore State Hospital in New York. These patients, whose serum cholesterol levels were above 240 mg. %, did not receive any other type of treatment known to have any effect on serum cholesterol, except 30½ fluid ounces of mineral water daily in three divided doses. The treatment continued for 30 days. At the end of two weeks, the average decrease of serum cholesterol was 9.9 mg. %. At the conclusion of the study, the average decrease was 23.8 mg. %.

A Hungarian doctor, O. Schulhof, M.D., made a study of the spa therapies and reported that, "Besides the psychological effects produced by the changed environment and the complex effect of various treatments, we still attribute importance to the specific effect of the mineral water." Dr. Schulhof said that it has been demonstrated that mineral water is actually absorbed through the skin during bathing. Mineral waters have been shown to have a beneficial effect on the connective tissues as well as on the immunological and healing powers of the body.

I have a firsthand experience with the value of mineral waters. During several years, I directed a biological clinic at a hot mineral spring spa in Mexico. We used mineral waters for bathing as well as for drinking. We have seen many striking examples of recovery from a multitude of acute and chronic conditions. I can agree with Dr. Schulhof that besides the complex effect of fasting, diet, and other therapies, I still attribute the remarkable results, at least in part, to the specific effect of mineral water.

Extensive studies in Europe and the United States showed that wherever people drink hard water (naturally heavily mineralized water) they have less heart disease, less tooth decay, less hardening of the arteries, and less diabetes than those who live in areas where soft water is used. Striking evidence comes from Monroe County, Florida, where the water supply was suddenly changed from rain water, with a hardness of .5 parts per million, to deep well water with a hardness 400 times greater. The death rate from heart disease and blood vessel diseases dropped from the 500-700 range to the 200-300 level within four years after the increase in water hardness (*Journal of American Dietetic Association*, Vol. 62., June 1973., p. 631).

I have stressed the danger of drinking soft, and especially distilled water in several of my books. *Are You Confused?* contains a chapter, "The Water Controversies," where I presented ample evidence that prolonged use of distilled water can be extremely harmful, and that minerals in hard water should form an essential part of our mineral nutrition. In spite of this, many people, still confused and brainwashed by some books and pamphlets on the subject, continue to drink distilled water, thereby damaging their health and shortening their lives.

Seawater — Mineral Gold Mine

Those who live close to the ocean can benefit from the rejuvenating and health-restoring effects of seawater minerals by frequent bathing in salt water, and also by drinking it.

Seawater is extremely rich in beneficial minerals. One or two tablespoons of pure seawater a day can be used internally as a mineral supplement. Some health food stores now sell purified seawater.

Minerals from the sea are also absorbed through the skin and through the inhaled mineral-rich air by the seashore. Make every effort to spend your holiday by the sea. In addition to providing the usual benefits of cold water bathing, salt water and salt air will recharge your system with health-restoring and rejuvenating minerals.

Juice Fasting

Perhaps the greatest contribution the Germans have given to the art and science of maintaining good health and enjoying long life is the development of the newest and most effective form of fasting — JUICE FASTING.

Fasting is not a German discovery, of course. It has been practiced throughout medical history, even before the advent of organized medicine. In fact, fasting is the oldest therapeutic method known to man. But, until just a few decades ago, the only form of fasting employed by practitioners was a traditional, classic form of fasting —a pure water fast—the abstinence from all foods and drinks with the exception of pure water. Some American practitioners and health clinics still employ this anti-quated form of fasting.

In Europe, and particularly in Germany, a few pioneers of biological medicine began experimenting with a different form of fasting. The result was that now the traditional water fast is never employed in any of the spas and clinics in Europe. It is replaced with the juice fast, or *Rohsafte-Kur*, which all the leading fasting authorities in Germany have found to be superior to water fasting—more effective in healing disease and bringing about a more thorough cleansing and rejuvenation of the tissues.*

The scientific justification of the superiority of juice fasting is based on the following physiological facts:

1. The main causes of disease and aging are to be found in the derangement of normal processes of cell metabolism and cell regeneration. The accumulation of toxins and metabolic waste products interferes with the nourishment of the cells and slows down cell regeneration and new cell building. When the normal metabolic processes become deranged (due to nutritional deficiencies, sluggish digestion and elimination, sedentary life, and overeating) and the process of cell nourishment, replacement, and rebuilding slows down, your body starts to grow old, its resistance to disease will diminish, and various ills will start to appear. Keep in mind that only about half of your cells are in the peak of development, vitality and working condition. One fourth are usually in the process of development and growth, and the other fourth in the process of breaking down or dying. The healthy life processes and perpetual youth-

---

*) One of the originators of juice fasting is Dr. Eugene Heun, M.D., Ph.D. Other leading juice fast specialists in Germany are Dr. Otto Buchinger, Jr. and Dr. Werner Zabel.

fulness are maintained when there is perfect balance in this process of cell breakdown and replacement. If the cells are breaking down and dying at a faster rate than the new cells are built, the process of aging will begin to set in. Also, it is of vital importance that the aging and dying cells are decomposed and eliminated as soon as possible. Quick and effective elimination of dead cells stimulates the building and growth of new cells.

Here is where juice fasting comes in as the most effective way to restore your health and rejuvenate your body. During a juice fast, the process of elimination of the dead and dying cells is speeded up, and the building of new cells is accelerated and stimulated.

2. During a juice fast, the eliminative and cleansing capacity of the eliminative organs — lungs, liver, kidneys, bowels and skin — is greatly increased and masses of accumulated metabolic wastes and toxins are quickly expelled.

3. Juice fasting exerts a normalizing, stabilizing and rejuvenating effect on all the vital physiological, nervous and mental functions. The nervous system is rejuvenated; mental powers are improved; glandular chemistry and hormonal secretions are stimulated.

4. Vitamin deficiencies and mineral imbalance in the tissues are the main causes of diminished oxygenation of cells, which leads to disease and premature aging of cells. Raw juices are rich in vitamins, enzymes, minerals, and trace elements. These are easily assimilated directly into the bloodstream and help to restore biochemical and mineral balance in the tissues and cells, and, thus, help to speed recovery and rejuvenate the tissues.

5. Overacidity in the tissues is one of the main causes of disease. Especially during fasting, blood and tissues contain large amounts of acids as a result of autolysis, or self-digestion. Raw juices provide an alka-

line surplus, which is extremely important for the proper acid-alkaline balance.

6. According to Dr. Ralph Bircher, raw juices contain an as yet unidentified factor which stimulates what he calls a "micro-electric tension" in the body, and is responsible for the cells' ability to absorb nutrients from the bloodstream and effectively excrete metabolic wastes.

Thus, raw juices are of particular importance when you fast for the regeneration and rejuvenation of your body. Juice fasting will help to break down and dispose of old, dying cells, revitalize the active cells, and accelerate the building of young vital cells.

Here's what Dr. Ragnar Berg, one of the world's greatest authorities on nutrition and biochemistry, said about the superiority of juice fasting over water fasting:

"During fasting, the body burns up and excretes huge amounts of accumulated wastes. We can help this cleansing process by drinking alkaline juices instead of water while fasting. I have supervised many fasts, and made extensive tests of fasting patients, and I am convinced that drinking alkaline-forming fruit and vegetable juices instead of water during fasting will increase the healing effect of fasting. The elimination of uric acid and other inorganic acids will be accelerated. And sugars in juices will strengthen the heart. Juice fasting is, therefore, the best form of fasting."

The foremost fasting authority in the world today, Dr. Otto H.F. Buchinger, Jr., M.D., has directed and supervised over 100,000 fasts in his clinic (more than any other doctor in the world). He told me that he employs only juice fasting, because, in his experience, "fasting on fresh raw juices of fruits and vegetables, plus vegetable broths and herb teas, results in much faster recovery from disease and more effective cleansing and rejuvenation of the tissues than does the water fast."

I have studied various methods of fasting for several decades in many countries. Among my teachers in biological medicine and fasting I am proud to count Are Waerland, Ragnar Berg, Werner Zabel, and Otto Buchinger, Jr. — all leading fasting authorities. I have also had personal experience with directing and supervising the fasting of hundred of patients, and observing the results of various fasting methods on specific conditions. I can testify that juice fasting is, indeed, superior to water fasting. It is the best, safest, and most effective healing method I know. Juice fasting not only accomplishes a physiological rejuvenation and revitalization of your body, but also has a profound effect on your mind and mental faculties. It stimulates and sharpens mental and aesthetic perception and increases your spiritual awareness.

Juice fasting—this modern, scientific health-restoring and rejuvenating miracle—will recharge, renew, and rejuvenate your whole personality—physically, sexually, mentally, and spiritually.

(For a complete description of the philosophy and mechanics of juice fasting, and for detailed instructions for a do-it-yourself fast, see *How to Keep Slim, Healthy and Young with Juice Fasting*, available at all leading health food stores, or from HEALTH PLUS, Publishers, P.O. Box 22001, Phoenix, Arizona 85028).

Warning from the Publisher:

There are several fasting clinics in the United States which continue to employ the outmoded water fast without enemas, and laying in bed throughout the whole length of fast. Such fasts can be extremely dangerous and can lead to serious health disorders including severe kidney damage. We advise those who consider undergoing a supervised fast to inquire as to which fasting method the practitioner or clinic uses before making a commitment. Those who wish to find a doctor or a clinic that uses a juice fasting method, as described by Dr. Airola in this chapter, may send a self-addressed stamped envelope and request to: International Academy of Biological Medicine, P.O. Box 31313, Phoenix, Arizona 85046. They will send a Directory of Doctors and Clinics free of charge.

Health and Longevity Secrets from

BULGARIA

As I mentioned in the first chapter, Ilja Metchnikoff, the famous Russian scientist, revolutionized medical thinking on aging when he published his famous theory on the prolongation of life by preventing autotoxemia due to colonic putrefaction and the development of toxins in the colon.

Metchnikoff made studies of the Bulgarian eating habits and became convinced that their exceptional longevity is the result of their special diet. It is well known that Bulgarians consume more soured milk in the form of yogurt and kefir than do people of any other nation. Metchnikoff claimed that the generous and continuous use of soured milk products, such as yogurt, kefir, and acidophilus milk, helps to prevent putrefaction in the colon and the consequent autotoxemia or self-poisoning, thus, improving health and prolonging life.

Bulgarians seem to be living proof of Dr. Metchnikoff's theory. They are healthy and tall people — the tallest people in Europe. They also live longer than most other people on earth. They have more centenarians — people who live to be 100 or more—than any other civilized nation. According to statistics they have 1,600 centenarians for every one million people, as compared to only seven persons 100 years or older per million in the United States.

Bulgarians are known to retain the characteristics of youth to an advanced age. The virility of their "old" men is legendary.

There is extensive literature to support yogurt as a longevity food. We must keep in mind, however, that the yogurt consumed by most Bulgarian centenarians is not made from cow's milk, but from sheep's or goat's milk. It is well known that the health-building and youth-preserving qualities of sheep's and goat's milk are superior to those of cow's milk. The protein and mineral composition of goat's or sheep's milk is closer to that of human milk than is cow's milk. Raw or fermented goat's milk contains anti-cancer and anti-arthritis factors, which may account in part for its life-prolonging property.

Yogurt is not the only Bulgarian secret for a long, healthy life. My study of Bulgarian centenarians and their living and eating habits revealed that they adhere to many other health-building and rejuvenating living habits:

- Most of them are predominantly lacto-vegetarians. That is, their diet consists mostly of locally-grown and freshly stone-ground whole grains (especially barley), and fresh vegetables and fruits from their own gardens. They eat very little meat. Only about 3 or 4 percent of all centenarians that I studied eat meat regularly.
- Most Bulgarian centenarians are beekeepers and use natural, unprocessed pollen-rich honey in their diet.
- They consume lots of fermented foods — especially sauerkraut. As you have seen in the previous chapter, fermented foods help to prevent and cure many diseases, and, thus, prolong life.
- Almost all Bulgarian centenarians eat raw, fresh

(not salted and roasted) sunflower seeds as an essential part of their diet.

- They live "close to nature," following nature's rhythm in working, eating, and sleeping; they are usually poor to the extent that they cannot afford to overeat; they are always engaged in hard physical work; they are friendly, contented, and have no inordinate ambitions or jealousy.

Here we have it: a Bulgarian blueprint for a happy, healthy, and long life. No fancy secrets, tricky diets or life-extension drugs — just simple common sense natural foods, and wholesome stress-free country living. But don't be deceived by its apparent simplicity. The factors mentioned—a lacto-vegetarian diet, yogurt, honey, sunflower seeds, fermented foods, and moderate eating— are all scientifically proven potent factors in preventing premature aging and prolonging life.

5

Health and Longevity Secrets from

RUSSIA

Russians are far ahead of other countries in research on longevity. While in the United States the preoccupation with rejuvenation or attempts to prolong one's life are considered by most scientists to be an oddity at best, if not inane health-faddist notions, in the USSR the prolongation of life is a legitimate science. There are several research institutes on longevity financed by the government. Extensive research has been going on at these centers for decades. Russian medical scientists consider the prevention of disease and prolongation of life their ultimate goals. Well-known Russian physiologist, Tarkhanov, wrote:

"The time will come when it will be a disgrace for a man to die less than 100 years old."

One of the Soviet scientists engaged in research on longevity is Olga Lepeshinskaya. In her book, *Life, Age and Longevity*, she states that the normal life span of human beings should not be less than *150 years*, if they would observe the elementary laws of health. Everyone who feels old before he reaches 100, she says, is suffering from premature old age. She claims that premature aging, like other diseases, can be prevented.

It can also be successfully treated after it appears. How? Here's her recipe:

- Sound, simple, natural nutrition.
- Plenty of physical work, recreation, and rest.
- Cheerful, optimistic outlook on life.

We must agree that this simple program will "work" for anyone who will conscientiously apply it in his life.

Of the many rejuvenation secrets that the Russians have discovered, I will bring to you a few of the more important ones. I have made extensive travels and studies in Russia, and I can assure you that Russians are, indeed, superior to us as far as health and longevity are concerned. They are known for their endurance and stamina. They have seven times more centenarians per million than the United States. In Abkhazia, the Russian province in Caucasus where many of the centenarians live, the average life expectancy for both men and women is over 90 years!

Pollen-Rich Honey

The discovery of pollen-rich honey as a life prolonger was made in the course of research in one of the Longevity Institutes in Russia. The famed Russian scientist, biologist, and experimental botanist, Dr. Nicolai Tsitsin, was engaged in research on longevity. The aim of his inquiry was to find ways of prolonging human life.

"We decided to send letters to 200 people claiming to be over 100 years old with the request to answer the following three questions: what was their age; how had they earned their living most of their lives; and what had been their principal food."

Dr. Tsitsin received 150 replies to his 200 letters.

"We made a very interesting discovery. The answers showed that a large number of them were beekeepers. And *all of them*, without exception, said that their principal food had always been honey!"

But, as sensational as this discovery was, this was not all!

"We found," continued Dr. Tsitsin, "that in each case, it wasn't really honey these people ate, but the waste matter in the bottom of the honey containers. Because most beekeepers were poor, they sold all of the pure honey, keeping only the 'dirty residue' for themselves."

After a series of laboratory tests, Dr. Tsitsin discovered that the "dirty residue" of the honey was not a dirt at all, but almost pure honey-bee pollen, which all honey is normally "contaminated" with. Thus, Tsitsin discovered one of the most important longevity secrets of Russian centenarians—pollen-rich, natural, unheated, unfiltered, and unprocessed honey!

Of course, the fact that honey and bee pollen are age-retarding and rejuvenating foods isn't really a Russian discovery; they have been considered such since time immemorial. Cave paintings from the Neolithic age show illustrations of honeycombs being gathered for food. Honey has been found in 3,000-year-old Egyptian pyramids. Pythagoras, the great Greek scientist, 600 B.C., recommended honey for health and long life. Many other Greek philosophers claimed that bee pollen held the secret of eternal youth. The original Olympic athletes used unstrained pollen-rich honey for extra energy and vitality. Throughout the ages, honey and pollen have been regarded as *ambrosia* — divine foods with age-retarding and life-prolonging properties.

The miraculous rejuvenative property of pollen-rich honey is attributed to the fact that pollen is nature's own propagator of life. It is the male germ cell of the plant kingdom. Pollen, in addition to all known water-soluble vitamins — including the hard-to-find B_{12} — and a rich supply of minerals, trace elements, and enzymes, contains *deoxiribosides* and *sterines*, plus *steroid* hormone substances. Pollen also contains a *gonadotrophic hormone*, a plant hormone which is similar to the pituitary hormone, *gonadotrophin*, which stimulates sex glands. During the last two decades, much research has been done, mostly in Russia and Sweden, to uncover the medicinal and rejuvenative value of bee pollen and honey. Both have been found to be miraculous rejuvenators and life-prolongators largely by improving general health, preventing disease, increasing the power of the body's own immunological mechanism, and stimulating and rejuvenating glandular activity.

There is a huge amount of research available on bee pollen, which shows that it is an effective treatment of such varied disorders as prostate troubles, hemorrhoids, asthma, allergies, digestive disorders and intestinal putrefaction, chronic bronchitis, multiple sclerosis, gastric ulcers, arthritis, hay fever — and, of course, the symptoms of aging.

I have mentioned previously the rejuvenative and health-building property of fermented, lactic-acid foods. French researcher, Dr. Remy Chauvin, reports that bee pollen seems to have an anti-putrefactive factor similar to that of fermented or lactic-acid foods. Pollen destroys harmful bacteria in the intestines and improves assimilation of nutrients and elimination of waste matter.

Honey is, of course, an undisputed health-building and age-retarding miracle food. More than any other food (with the possible exception of the next secret — garlic and onions), it fulfills Hippocrates' requirement for the ideal food: i.e., "Let your food be your medicine — let your medicine be your food."

It has been demonstrated that honey:

- increases calcium retention (so important for staying younger longer);

- increases hemoglobin (red blood cell) count and can help prevent or cure nutritional anemia (it contains iron and copper);
- has a beneficial effect on healing processes in such conditions as arthritis, colds, poor circulation, constipation, liver and kidney disorders, weak heart action, bad complexion, and insomnia;
- is rich in aspartic acid, an important amino acid which is involved in the rejuvenation processes, particularly in the rejuvenation of sex glands.

Now you can understand why pollen-rich honey is such an important health and longevity factor in the diet of all Russian and Bulgarian centenarians. Pollen and honey have, indeed, age-retarding, health-building, and life-prolongating properties.

It is difficult to obtain "pollen-contaminated" natural honey in the United States. Most honey sold in supermarkets is filtered, heated, and refined — and free from pollen! Health food stores sell unfiltered honey, which contains some pollen. However, honey-bee pollen is now available in pure form at all better health food stores. In your stay-younger-longer diet, take 1 to 2 tbsp. of pollen every day. And, replace all sugar — including so-called brown sugar — with natural honey.

Garlic and Onions

At the end of the Second World War, when American troops finally confronted the Russian troops, some American soldiers discovered that many Russian soldiers had their pockets filled with onions and garlic, and judging from the odor, they made good use of them. For several years, the Russian Army fought on a near-starvation diet because of a severe food shortage. But two things always seemed to be in good supply: garlic and onions. In addition to buckwheat porridge and black rye bread, garlic and onions comprised the Russian Army's staple ration.

While traveling in Russia, I enjoyed stopping at the villages and studying the life in the agricultural collectives, their methods of cultivation, preferred crops, etc. In addition to the collectively owned fields, each family was allowed to have a large garden of their own, where they could grow anything they wished for their own use or for sale on the public market. I have found that two vegetables completely dominated these gardens: cabbage (for sauerkraut) and onions!

Russian electrobiologist, Professor Gurwitch, discovered that garlic and onions emit a peculiar type of ultra-violet radiation called mitogenetic radiation. This radiation—the Gurwitch rays—has the property of stimulating cell growth and activity and has a rejuvenating effect on all body functions.

A great amount of scientific research has been done in various countries on the therapeutic properties of garlic and onions. Dr. A.I. Virtanen, Finnish Nobel Prize Winner, discovered 14 *new* beneficial substances in onions. Russian, Japanese, German, French, English, and American researchers have successfully used garlic to treat such varied conditions as high or low blood pressure, common colds, intestinal worms, cough, asthma, whooping cough, intestinal putrefaction, dysentery, gastrointestinal disorders, gas, tuberculosis, and diabetes. American research has shown that garlic is a powerful agent against tumor formation in cancer. It has also been found to be an effective agent in preventing pneumonia.

Russian researchers discovered that garlic has antibiotic properties. They often refer to garlic as "Russian penicillin." Russian medical clinics and hospitals use garlic extensively—mostly in the form of volatile extracts that are vaporized and inhaled.

I have found in my own practice that the most dramatic therapeutic use of garlic is, perhaps, in the treatment of high blood pressure. Almost without exception, blood pressure can be reduced in two weeks by 30-40 mm. by nothing but garlic therapy—by including generous quantities of raw garlic in the diet. High blood pressure is, of course, one of the causes of heart disease — our greatest killer. The fact that garlic has such a beneficial effect on reducing blood pressure makes it an important life-prolongator. By counter-acting intestinal putrefaction and improving assimilation of the essential nutrients from the intestines, garlic and onions improve health and prolong life. Not to mention the fact that garlic and onions also are most delicious foods!

Odor? Well, why not just do like Russians and Italians do: eat and enjoy; let the others worry about our odors! Or, take Kyolic (see Chapter 7)!

Buckwheat

During my meeting with one of the leading Russian scientists in the field of preventative medicine and longevity, the question came up regarding Russia's low incidence of cardiovascular disease and heart attacks. The Russian scientist said:

"We have a relatively low incidence of high blood pressure and cardiovascular diseases, and we attribute this in part to our regular eating of such foods as garlic and buckwheat. Buckwheat supplies *rutin*, a bioflavonoid, which we have found to have a blood-pressure-reducing property, and a beneficial effect on the circulatory system."

Buckwheat, mostly in the form of a hot porridge, which they call *kasha*, is really the Russian national food. Wherever I've traveled in Russia, I have seen people eating kasha almost every day of their lives.

Kasha is served to all the personnel in the Russian Army several times a week, mostly with sunflower seed oil.

Buckwheat is an extremely nutritious cereal containing complete proteins, vitamins, and minerals — especially manganese and magnesium. It is low in sodium and very rich in potassium. Rutin in buckwheat makes it a very important age-retarding food, as circulation problems and cardiovascular disorders are at the root of the many aging processes. The proteins in buckwheat are of very high quality, comparable in biological value to proteins in meat and milk, as shown recently by a study of the U.S. Department of Agriculture.

If you wish to try this famous Russian longevity food, here is the recipe and instructions. Buckwheat grains can be bought at most health food stores.

KASHA
(Buckwheat cereal)

1 cup whole, raw (not roasted) buckwheat grains
2 to 2½ cups of water

Bring water to a boil. Stir the buckwheat into the boiling water and let boil for 2 to 3 minutes. Turn heat to low and simmer for 15 to 20 minutes, stirring occasionally. When all the water is absorbed, remove from the stove and let stand for another 15-30 minutes. Kasha must never be mushy. Serve hot or warm.

Russians eat kasha with sunflower seed oil, butter or flaxseed oil. Some children prefer it with milk and honey. I love it with a little cold-pressed virgin olive oil. If seasoning is desired, add a little sea salt to the cooking water.

Another way to cook kasha is the way Russians cook it in the country. Mix buckwheat grains in boiling water and place the covered stainless steel, stoneware, or other heat-proof pot (never aluminum) in an oven heated to 200° F. Leave for 3 to 4 hours (for example, make it in the morning and eat it for lunch). Delicious! Nutritious! And it will help keep you younger longer!

Other Longevity Secrets from Russia

In addition to pollen-rich honey, garlic and onions, and buckwheat, here are a few other health and longevity secrets from Russia:

1. Russians eat enormous quantities of raw sunflower seeds and use unrefined cold-pressed sunflower oil. Sunflower oil is rich in vitamin E and essential fatty acids, the deficiency of which is definitely linked with premature aging. Sunflower seeds are also an excellent source of complete protein, B vitamins, and minerals — especially zinc, which plays an important role in the growth and maturity of the gonads, the male sex glands, and also is vitally linked with the health of the prostate gland. Zinc has been pointed out as an active agent in most so-called virility foods, such as oysters, raw nuts, sea foods, onions, eggs, pumpkin seeds, etc.

2. Russians, like Germans, eat lots of fermented lactic-acid foods: sourdough bread, sauerkraut, dill pickles, and soured milks, like kefir, kumis, and plain clabbered milk. All these foods, as we have shown earlier, have a health-promoting and life-prolongating effect.

3. Russians eat more natural, unprocessed foods than we do. A very few chemical additives are allowed in food processing, and all artificial colorings and flavorings are totally prohibited. Artificial colorings and flavorings are extremely harmful. Recent studies show that they are the main cause of the growing ranks of overactive, or hyperkinetic, children in this country.

American children are fed huge amounts of artificial colorings and flavorings, which they get from soft drinks, processed cereals, and most other foods, including baby foods. Most travelers to Russia have remarked on the well-behaved, well-mannered, contented, and "quiet" Russian children.

4. Russians eat very little meat compared to Americans. Theirs is a comparatively low-protein diet, and most of their proteins are from vegetable and grain sources. Only 25.5% of their protein intake is acquired from animal sources (in the U.S. — 71%). As I will show you in the chapter on Hunza, over-consumption of animal proteins is one of the surest ways to fall victim of many so-called diseases of civilization, including cancer, and shorten your life.

Health and Longevity Secrets from

ROMANIA

On one of my frequent research trips to Europe, in 1968, I met the famous Romanian doctor, Professor Ana Aslan, M.D., of Bucharest. Dr. Aslan discovered the so-called *Gerovital* therapy—the rejuvenation therapy also known as KH-3, GH3, procaine, or novocaine therapy. At 70, Dr. Aslan looked like she could be in her late fifties. Her face was quite free from wrinkles, and even the skin on her arms was perfectly smooth and firm as on a younger person. She was good advertising for her rejuvenation discovery. Now, at 83, she still looks younger than her age and continues to be extremely active.

About 35 years ago, Dr. Aslan discovered, quite accidentally, that procaine, commonly used mild anesthetic agent, has an age-retarding property. She injected specially designed doses of procaine — which she named H-3 — into patients showing signs of degeneration and premature aging. She observed that stiff, immobile joints became flexible, pain disappeared, and the patients gained new energy and vitality. Since then, Dr. Aslan has improved her original H-3 formula and now uses a potassium and benzoic acid-enriched formula called Gerovital, which she claims has been demonstrated in tests in Italy and the U.S.A. to be superior to pure procaine.

Gerovital has been used in Romania for over 30 years, and thousands upon thousands of people from Europe and other countries travel to Dr. Aslan's Geriatric Institute in Bucharest to receive Gerovital treatments in modern government-owned clinics under the supervision of dozens of Aslan-trained doctors. Dr. Aslan said that well over 100,000 people have been treated at her Institute.

I have seen many of those who have received treatment at the Bucharest Institute, and also have myself supervised dozens of patients who took KH-3 (the trademark of German-made oral Gerovital) at my clinic in Mexico.* I have seen many rather enthusiastic patients who claimed that KH-3 had a revitalizing and rejuvenating effect on them. I have also seen rather dramatic improvements in some patients with chronic degenerative conditions. This is the reason I decided to share with you my knowledge of, and my experience with, Gerovital, although it is not a natural treatment by any means, but a drug. This is not a recommendation or endorsement, just a passing-on of information. Since procaine is not a nutrient, herb, or natural substance, I cannot, being a naturopathic physician, give it my unreserved endorsement. On the other hand, this substance is claimed to be completely harmless and is sold and endorsed for use by the medical governments of many countries, including Switzerland, Holland, Belgium, England, East and West Germany, Romania, and Mexico.

According to Dr. Aslan, the aging processes start when the body's ability to produce new cells and to

---

*) I am referring to my Biological Medical Clinic in Guadalajara in the late 60's and early 70's. I have no clinics or practice at present.

replenish or repair the old ones is diminished. Gerovital helps the body to regenerate new cell production, which is the reason for its rejuvenative effect.

In Bucharest Institute, Gerovital (GH3) is usually administered intramuscularly three times a week for four weeks. The treatment can be repeated after a pause of two to four weeks. The reports from the Aslan Institute are that Gerovital-treated patients experience reduction in cholesterol levels; normalized blood pressure; improvement in memory; disappearance of wrinkles, dryness of the skin, and other visible symptoms of aging; increase in muscular strength; and noticeable improvement in patients suffering from anxiety and depression. Some patients regrew hair in bald areas. Occasionally, pigmentation was restored to graying hair.

Does Gerovital really work? Or is it just another of a growing number of useless "youth drugs"? The AMA has declared GH3 useless for anything other than a local anesthetic. However, a growing number of independent researchers claim that Gerovital may be effective in the treatment of symptoms of aging; if it does not prevent, it may at least postpone some of the common degenerative diseases, and thus, postpone the aging processes and prolong life. But, how does Gerovital work?

Two American studies have shed some light on the possible reasons for the alleged rejuvenation properties of Gerovital. Alfred Sapsa of UCLA, and M. David McFarlane of the University of Southern California, tested GH3 and found it to be a MAO inhibitor. MAO (monoamine oxidase) is an enzyme that breaks down various amines that are formed in the body. Some of these amines come from foods, some are produced by the body for various vital functions. For example, the body under stress may produce epinephrine (adrenaline) or norepinephrine. MAO destroys (deaminates) these stimulators when they are no longer needed or when an excess is present. It is generally believed that MAO levels tend to rise with age, and, because of that, old people are often deficient in these stimulants and neurotransmittors. This depresses the activity of the nervous system and the brain, and causes anxiety, depression, and loss of interest in life that often accompanies old age. Thus, the MAO inhibiting property of Gerovital may be responsible for the alleged increased energy, decreased depression, and the feeling of youthful vitality that Gerovital-treated patients seem to enjoy.

Another clue to the effectiveness of Gerovital in halting the aging processes comes from a study by B.M. Zuckerman at the University of Massachusetts Laboratory of Experimental Biology. He found that GH3 retards the formation of lipofuscin (in studies with nematodes) and inhibits the development of liver spots (lipofuscin deposits) in humans. It is generally believed that the accumulation of lipofuscin (the aging pigment in the body cells) contributes to the accelerated aging processes.

Some studies now in progress indicate that Gerovital also may have a strengthening effect on cell membranes — another possible pathway towards the prevention of premature aging.

Until very recently, Gerovital was not allowed to be sold in the United States because of the FDA ban. Now, however, it is allowed to be sold in the state of Nevada only. There is an American company in Nevada that has allegedly obtained exclusive rights from the Romanian Government to import and distribute the drug in the United States.

In larger Mexican cities, even on the American border, major pharmaceutical stores sell KH-3, a German-manufactured oral equivalent of GH3. It is a special catalyst combination formula which contains hematoporphyrine, an active factor obtained from hemoglobin. It is claimed that hematoporphyrine is an effective synergist of protein, and that it enhances procaine's rejuvenative effect. But the catalyst, hematoporphyrine, by itself, also effects an improvement in the vital areas of cellular metabolism and glandular functions within the organs in a biological manner. It also improves the functions of the sexual glands. KH-3 is usually taken one capsule a day for three to five months. Dr. Aslan recommends Gerovital only to persons over 40 years of age.

Notes:
1. By giving you this information on Gerovital, I do not endorse or recommend it: I only report objectively what I know about it.
2. Please, do not confuse GH3 (Gerovital), the original Aslan's procaine-based product, with many inferior products currently on the market that bear names similar to Gerovital or GH3, but which contain no procaine. Read labels carefully.
3. I do not sell Gerovital and am not connected with it, or Dr. Aslan, in any way. Perhaps I should mention in this connection that I do not sell vitamins, food supplements, or any of the other products mentioned in this book, nor do I own or operate any health food stores.

Health and Longevity Secrets from

JAPAN

Of all my worldwide travels, my extended tour of Japan was one of the highlights. Ironically, I was invited to Japan to present several lectures to professionals and the public on the latest European and American developments in the sciences of nutrition and holistic health. In the concluding address which I gave during the farewell banquet in my honor, I surprised the audience (and even myself) when I said:

"You will be better off if you forget everything I have said in my lectures. You have nothing to learn from America in the matters of health and nutrition. Your own traditional eating patterns are far superior to anything that the West can offer you. I am convinced that I have learned more from you regarding nutrition and health than you have learned from me. So here is my parting advice: Stay away from American nutritionists — they can only confuse you and lead you on the wrong path. You are now enjoying much better health than Americans do; and you can give credit for it to your own superior eating and living habits. So, stick to your own traditional nutrition, eat lots of seaweeds and soba, shun all the Western dietary influences like the plague, and do not let American fast-food conglomerates and ice cream parlors into your country."

I have learned many health and longevity secrets from the health-oriented Japanese, such as their traditional hot baths, delicious and super-nutritious buckwheat soba, fermented soy foods, etc. But, in terms of importance, the generous use of seaweeds in the Japanese diet is, perhaps, their number one health and longevity secret.

SEAWEED

The traditional Japanese diet contains a large percentage of seaweed. In some parts of Japan, as much as one fourth of the daily diet is made up of seaweed in various forms. The Japanese make soups, noodles, casseroles, and other dishes with seaweed.

There are many kinds of edible seaweed. In England and Ireland, the most popular kind is *dulse*, the crisp and tender leaves of which are called "sea lettuce." In Scotland, Norway, and Iceland, a seaweed called *porphyra*, which "looks like spinach, and tastes like oysters," is commonly eaten. In the United States, seaweed called *kelp* has been extremely popular among health food advocates.

In the Japanese diet, there are many kinds of seaweeds. The most commonly-eaten seaweed is a large-leafed brown seaweed similar to that from which the familiar granulated kelp is made. The Japanese are among the most vigorous, industrious, and healthy people in the world. Until very recently, white bread, sugar, ice cream, soft drinks, milk, meat, etc., were virtually unknown in Japan, and the Japanese enjoyed excellent health and one of the best records of longevity in the East. Their diet was largely vegetarian, with the addition of fish, but almost total absence of meat. One of the staples in their diet was, and still is, seaweed, or kelp.

Why do I place kelp as one of the most important health secrets? Because kelp is a true wonder food of nature, loaded with vital substances not available in any other food.

Kelp is extremely rich in natural iodine, which is essential for the endocrine glands, especially the thyroid. Iodine deficiency can disrupt normal thyroid functions and cause diminished hormone production. Thyroid hormone, thyroxine, is largely responsible for your youthful appearance, for your sex appeal, sexual vigor, and libido. Very few foods contain iodine, as most soils, especially in the United States, are deficient in this mineral.

Finnish geologist, Professor V. Auer, warned that man's health and reproductive capacity is in danger because food from depleted soils lacks the minerals and trace elements which are vital for health. For thousands of years, minerals from tilled soils have been washed with the rains and rivers into the sea. These minerals are taken up by the seaweed plants. Seaweed returns to man's diet what soils can no longer supply. The chemical composition of seawater is virtually identical to that of human blood. Thus, seawater contains *all* the minerals and trace elements necessary to build and sustain health.

Dr. W.A.P. Black, of the British Nutrition Society, says that "Seaweed contains all the elements that have so far been shown to play an important part in the physiological processes of man." The vitamin C content of seaweed is very high — sometimes higher than in oranges. Seaweed has been the only source of vitamin C for many Eskimo tribes and has helped them to survive on an otherwise unhealthful diet. Kelp also contains vitamins B, A, E, K, D, and even B_{12}, which is seldom found in foods of vegetable origin. In addition to large amounts of such minerals as calcium, potassium, and chlorine, kelp contains trace minerals such as manganese, copper, silicon, boron, barium, lithium, strontium, zinc, and vanadium. Kelp is extremely rich in all these vital elements because it grows in an ideal environment, with no risk of depletion as it is constantly renewed by nature.

Seaweed is also an excellent source of high quality proteins, which are comparable in biological value to animal proteins.

Seaweed is an essential ingredient in one of the most famous Oriental aphrodisiacs — *Bird Nest Soup*. Bird nest soup is prepared from the nest of the sea-swallow. The secret of the aphrodisiac efficacy of bird nest soup is that swallows make their nests from seaweed plants which they glue together with fish spawn. Spawn is rich in phosphorus, and seaweed — with its storehouse of important minerals, particularly iodine — has a rejuvenative and stimulating effect on glandular activity, especially on the thyroid gland, which is responsible for sex drive and libido. Kelp aids in the formation of the thyroid hormone, thyroxine, which regulates the utilization of oxygen by all the cells of the body. Many researchers feel that insufficient oxygenation of cells is at the root of the aging processes. Thus, kelp, seaweeds, or bird nest soup may be the best fountains of youth yet!

Bird nest soup is served in all better Oriental restaurants in the United States, although it is prohibitively expensive. A less expensive and equally effective way to rejuvenate yourself is to learn from the Japanese and make seaweeds an essential part of your diet. Kelp is sold in all health food stores in tablet form or granules. It could be added to salads, soups, breads, or vegetable juices. It is an excellent substitute for salt ... which should be excluded from a health and longevity diet anyway, as you can see from the following.

SALT—A KILLER IN DISGUISE

Another important health and longevity secret that comes from Japan concerns salt.

The U.N. sponsored World Health Organization (WHO) reported recently from Japan that it has been statistically demonstrated that the frequency of cancer of the stomach in Japan is definitely related to the quantity of salt consumed by the natives in different areas. The more salt in the diet — the more stomach cancers. Thus, salt has been indicted as one of the proven carcinogens. In one particular coastal area of Japan, the incidence of cancer is ten times higher than in the rest of the country. Traditionally, natives of that area eat lots of heavily salted fish. They use excessive amounts of salt in the preparation of other foods as well.

It is significant, however, that only refined commercial salt has been shown to cause cancer. Where natives use kelp, seawater, or natural unrefined sea salt to season their foods, they enjoy excellent health and avoid stomach cancer.

Cancer is, of course, not the only thing that is caused by excessive consumption of salt. Although beneficial in small amounts, salt is extremely toxic in large doses, and is a contributing cause of such disorders as kidney problems, heart and blood vessel conditions, high blood pressure, rheumatic diseases, hair loss, and many skin disorders.

Americans eat far too much salt with their food. Research has revealed that the daily requirement of salt is between 0.2 and 0.6 grams. This amount of salt can easily be obtained from the natural foods you eat, provided that you eat predominantly raw, uncooked foods (as you should if you are interested in staying younger longer!). The average American consumes 10-15 grams of salt a day. In such amounts, salt becomes a dangerous poison, causing illness and shortening life.

In your stay-young diet, keep salt to an absolute minimum. If you use salt, use only natural, unrefined sea salt. Still better, use kelp liberally as a salt substitute. While white, refined salt is a life shortener, kelp is one of the best-proved health-building, life-prolonging foods.

KYOLIC

While in Japan, I uncovered another health and longevity secret, which is now widely available in the United States and Canada: Kyolic.

What is Kyolic? First, let me say that Kyolic is not a part of the traditional Japanese diet. It is a new health and longevity supplement developed by the ingenious and enterprising Japanese. Kyolic is a completely natural, odorless garlic preparation sold in three forms: liquid, capsule, and tablet. By a special fermentation process, which involves curing crushed, organically grown garlic in huge vats for twenty months without the use of heat or other processing, garlic loses its familiar odor and can be taken internally without resulting in any body or breath odor — even when taken in huge doses.

You read in Chapter 5 about some of the remarkable nutritional and medicinal properties of garlic. The format of this book will not allow me to go into as much detail as I would like to,* but let me just list here a few scientifically-proven properties of garlic:

---

*) Those who wish to study the garlic story in detail should read my book, *The Miracle of Garlic*. It is a fully documented treatise on the amazing medicinal and nutritional aspects of garlic.

- Garlic has a dilating effect on blood vessels and can reduce blood pressure dramatically.
- Garlic can prevent the development of athero-sclerosis and consequent heart disease.
- Garlic can lower the serum cholesterol levels and prevent the formation of plaques in arteries.
- Garlic raises the hemoglobin and red-cell count and can be effective in the treatment of anemia.
- Garlic extract, Kyolic, was shown to be "remark-ably effective" in treatment of patients with lumbago and arthritis.
- Garlic is one of the few completely harmless natural substances which are effective in the treatment of diabetes.
- Garlic strengthens the body's defenses against allergens and can be used effectively in the treatment of both allergy and hypoglycemia.
- Garlic has proven antibiotic properties. Russian studies show a noticeable inhibition of bacterial growth and accelerated healing processes after garlic administration.
- Garlic possesses antibacterial, antiviral, and anti-fungal properties.
- Garlic is one of the few effective treatments against herpes, both genital and other types.
- Garlic preparations have been used successfully against cancer, both in animal and human studies.
- Garlic is one of the richest natural sources of germanium, a trace mineral, which has been found to have both preventive and curative effects on cancer.
- Garlic is an excellent source of biologically-effec-tive selenium. The trace element selenium has a protective effect against the development of can-cer — specifically breast cancer — heart disease,

and premature aging. It is a powerful natural antioxidant and free-radical deactivator. Selenium also detoxifies mercury, as well as neutralizes many other carcinogenic substances in the body. Selenium is one of the proven life-prolongators.

- Garlic is a powerful detoxifier. Japanese studies show that garlic can neutralize most of the environmental poisons that enter our bodies with food, air, and water, and protect our bodies from their harmful effects.

- Garlic can protect us from the health-damaging effects of heavy metal poisons. Japanese and Russian studies show that garlic can effectively bind (chelate) such toxic metals as lead, mercury, and cadmium in our bodies, and help to excrete them safely from the system.

"Wow!" I hear you exclaiming. Isn't this an impressive list of the amazing health-promoting, disease-preventing, and life-extending properties of garlic?! And, this is only a partial list. Moreover, every property of garlic mentioned above is well documented by scientific references listed in my book, *The Miracle of Garlic.*

Perhaps this old English folk saying wasn't far off:

"Eat onions in March, and garlic in May —

Then the rest of the year, your doctor can play."

Now, if you are convinced that garlic should be a regular ingredient in your stay-young-and-healthy program, the question in your mind is: "How can I use garlic in our society of mouthwashes and deodorants? It may be okay in Italy, Russia, or Korea, but you just don't go around reeking of garlic in our culture. My marriage may be ruined, I may lose my job, and I certainly will never be able to come within six feet of anyone!"

That's where my Japanese health and longevity secret, Kyolic, comes into fore! You can now benefit from all the traditional amazing medicinal, therapeutic, and nutritional properties of garlic without social limitations and repercussions. Take 3-4 capsules of liquid Kyolic twice a day, or 2-3 tablets three times a day, and you will improve your health, help prevent disease, and live younger longer. Kyolic Super Formula 101 is my favorite Kyolic product. It is specially formulated to help protect against environmental toxins, especially against heavy metal poisons such as lead, mercury, and cadmium, to which we are all subjected in this age of universal pollution. Kyolic, the odor-free garlic product, is sold in most health food stores.

Health and Longevity Secrets from
HUNZA

Hunza, an isolated kingdom in the Himalayas, is known to be a country without disease. Hunza people are also known for their legendary longevity. Many live to be 110 and 125 years of age, and are strong, virile, and active as long as they live, retaining their youthful appearance far into advanced age. Their men have been known to sire children after they reached 100. The *average* life expectancy in Hunza is between 85 and 90 years!

Many investigators have tried to pin down the health and longevity secrets of the people of Hunza. The most authoritative and reliable information comes from Dr. Robert McCarrison who lived among them for seven years. Dr. McCarrison's conclusion was that the traditional diet of the Hunza people was, more than anything else, responsible for their extraordinary health and longevity. Many investigators and authors have visited Hunza since McCarrison, and each one expressed their conclusions as to the Hunzakuts' health and longevity secrets. One of the scientific investigators to study the health and longevity records of the Hunza people was my friend, Dr. Karl-Otto Aly, of Sweden. With a group of Swedish researchers, he stayed in Hunza for several weeks and made a thorough study of their health conditions, their living habits, and their nutrition patterns.

Most investigators point out that, in addition to the fact that the Hunza people live a life protected from such hazards of civilization as polluted air, water, and soil and refined, processed foods, the two most important factors in their unusual health and longevity are:

1. Their high-natural-carbohydrate, low-animal-protein diet.

2. The highly mineralized water they drink.

Let's look at these two most important health and longevity secrets from Hunza.

LOW-ANIMAL-PROTEIN DIET— HUNZA'S HEALTH AND LONGEVITY SECRET NUMBER ONE

Dr. Karl-Otto Aly, M.D., is one of the leading biologically and nutritionally oriented doctors in Europe. He is an internationally recognized authority on health and nutrition. In addition to being the director of a large and successful biological clinic in Sweden, he writes and travels extensively, lecturing on health and how it can be built and maintained.

Dr. Aly made an extensive study of the health conditions and the living habits of the Hunza people during his stay among them. He examined their birth and death records, spoke to the only physician who lives and practices in the country (who, according to the King of Hunza, "does not have much to do"), did physical examinations of the natives, and made many tests. Here's what Dr. Aly wrote after his return from Hunza:

"Their daily diet, even today, consists of natural, poison-free high quality foods, and is mostly vegetarian. The variety of vegetables and fruits guarantees their adequate supply of various minerals, vitamins, and proteins. The fact that Hunzakuts not only survived in their isolated, rugged mountains, but are enjoying such a high level of health and vitality on such a diet, speaks for its inherent superiority.

"According to today's scientific norms and recommendations, the diet of Hunzakuts is utterly protein-deficient, and even deficient in vitamin B_{12}. If we would believe today's orthodox nutritionists, the people of Hunza should have been dead circa 2,000 years ago, when they inhabited this isolated river valley and began eating their traditional low-animal-protein diet. But, apparently not knowing that modern science would not approve of their diet, they fared quite well for over 2,000 years. Just like a bumble-bee, which according to all statistical and aerodynamic calculations can't fly, but, being ignorant of the laws of aerodynamics and gravity, flies anyway! Not only did the people of Hunza survive with flying colors, but even today I could not discover a single case of protein deficiency (kwashiorkor), or anemia and nerve degeneration caused by a B_{12} deficiency."

We are living in an era of the high-protein craze. Some modern nutritionists and doctors, misled by erroneous conclusions of some 19th century scientists and by slanted research paid for by the meat and dairy industries, have been brainwashing us to believe that we must eat "lots of protein" if we wish to be healthy and live long. Disregarding all the empirical evidence to the contrary, they are telling us that not only do we need lots of protein — "the more the better" — but also that we must eat *animal* proteins — meat, fowl, eggs, milk, and fish—if we do not wish to succumb to most horrible diseases. Consequently, we have been filling ourselves up to our ears with proteins. Americans eat more protein than any other people. Also, according to statistics, the United States leads the world in most degenerative diseases, such as cancer, heart disease, arthritis, diabetes, and osteoporosis.

What's wrong? Could it possibly be that modern nutritional scientists have made a mistake? That, perhaps, a high-protein diet is not as "good for you" as they believed it would be? Perhaps their tales and scare stories about kwashiorkor and B_{12} deficiency anemia are not based on scientific facts, but on wishful thinking influenced by their own tastes?

The Hunza example, supported by a growing amount of new nutrition research from around the world, is contradicting and nullifying most of the claims made by the high-animal-protein diet advocates. The latest research shows that the high-protein theory was a myth; that most of our present beliefs and conclusions about proteins, our need for them, and their function in nutrition, *are wrong*. The most recently proven facts about protein, based on the most reliable and authoritative scientific research from independent sources, such as The Max Planck Institute in Germany, The Russian Institute for Nutritional Research, The International Society for Research on Civilization Diseases and Environment, and several universities in the U.S., show

- That our actual daily requirement of protein is much lower than was believed: not 200, 120, 80 or even 70 grams, as was advocated a decade ago, or 55 grams as recommended in the latest official tables, but 45 grams a day; even less if raw protein foods are used.

- That too much protein in the diet is extremely dangerous and can cause many health disturbances and serious diseases.

- That overconsumption of protein can cause a severe deficiency of calcium, magnesium, and vitamins B_6 and B_3.

- That too much animal protein in the diet contributes to such diseases as arthritis, osteoporosis, heart disease, and cancer. One of the by-products of meat metabolism, ammonia, is considered to be a strong carcinogen, and is now considered to be the number one cause of cancer of the colon.

- That too much protein can cause mental disorders, particularly schizophrenia.
- That too much animal protein in the diet, due to its excessive protein and fat content, leads to premature aging by causing biochemical imbalance, overacidity in tissues, intestinal putrefaction and constipation, degeneration of vital organs, and a build-up of free-radicals, which are now directly linked with accelerated aging processes.

Furthermore, the newest research has established the following extremely important facts, hitherto unknown to science:

1. That the commonly held belief that only animal proteins are complete, and that all vegetable proteins are incomplete, or lacking one or more essential amino acids, is false. Many vegetarian sources, such as soybeans, sunflower seeds, almonds, millet, buckwheat, sesame seeds, peanuts, potatoes, all sprouted seeds and grains, and all leafy green vegetables contain complete protein.

2. That some vegetable proteins are not only equal to, but they are actually *superior* in biological value to proteins of animal sources. For example, proteins in potatoes are biologically superior to proteins in meat, eggs, or milk (Max Planck Institute).

3. That raw proteins have higher biological values than cooked proteins. You need only about one-half the amount of proteins if you eat raw vegetable proteins instead of animal proteins, which are, as a rule, cooked.

High Protein Diet—a Sure Road to Premature Aging.

High-protein propagandists, meat and dairy industries, and protein supplement manufacturers use many tricks to induce you to eat huge amounts of protein. They say: you are made of protein; your hair, your nails, your enzymes, your organs, your hormones — all are made of protein. This is only a half-truth. Your hair, nails and vital organs are not made of protein only, but are made from minerals, trace elements, unsaturated and saturated fatty acids, lecithin ... *and* proteins!

Another method widely used by high-protein peddlers is preying on the public's gullibility and desire to "look and feel young." "Stay younger longer with lots of protein, especially meat!" The fact is that heavy meat eating is one of the surest ways to age before your time — physically, sexually, and mentally. The Hunza example illustrates clearly that *it is not a high-protein, but a low-protein diet which has the greatest potential for optimum health and long life.* Their average daily intake of protein is about 30 grams. Many other long-living people in the world—Russians, Yukatan Indians, Todas, Abkhazians, Vilcabamba inhabitants, and Bulgarians—eat low-protein diets. Hunzakuts eat meat once a month, at the most. According to a recent study of Dr. S. Magsood Ali, of Pakistan, only 1 percent of the Hunzakuts' protein intake is from animal sources. Bulgarians eat very little meat—perhaps 15-20 percent of the average American's consumption. In Russia, only 1½ percent of the total population are vegetarians, while 9 percent of all people who reach 100 years are vegetarians, which clearly shows the vegetarian diet's superiority as a longevity diet. Vilcabamba inhabitants in Ecuador show the largest number of centenarians of any place in the world—1,098 for every 100,000 people! According to Dr. Alexander Leaf, M.D., their average protein intake is 35-38 grams a day, and the total caloric intake is only 1,200 to 1,360 a day. They are almost 100 percent vegetarians. This is something to ponder for those who claim that lots of animal proteins in your diet will keep you younger longer. The opposite is true!

That a high-protein diet, particularly a high-animal-protein diet, is one of the main causes of senility and premature aging has been recently stressed by two leading European biochemists and doctors — Professor Ph. Schwarz, of Frankfurt University, and Dr. Ralph Bircher of Zurich, Switzerland. They reported that the aging processes are triggered by a substance called *amyloid*, a by-product of protein metabolism, which is deposited in connective tissues and causes tissue and organ degeneration. Amyloid, the aging-producing substance, contains a large percentage of the amino acids tryptophan and tyrosine, which are plentiful in animal proteins.

The connection between deposits of amyloid in the tissues and the degenerative diseases and aging processes in man has been known for a long time, but conveniently forgotten in this age of the high-protein fad. Famous German pathologist, Dr. Rudolf Virchow, suggested as early as 1854 that amyloid deposits cause degenerative changes and premature aging. Amyloidosis was produced in experimental animals by feeding them high-protein diets.

Here are some remarkable facts to ponder upon:

Fact number one: The consensus of medical experts is that amyloidosis, or high incidence of amyloid formation and deposit in connective tissues, nerve and brain cells, and other tissues of the body, triggers and accelerates the aging processes.

Fact number two: When researchers wish to test a new age-retarding drug on mice, they first induce in mice a state of amyloidosis, or excessive accumulation of amyloid in tissues, by feeding them a high-animal-protein diet.

Fact number three: Somehow, the same scientists are seemingly unable to draw a simple and logical conclusion from the two above-mentioned facts: that a high-animal-protein diet causes premature aging and shortened life by producing amyloidosis. Unperturbed, they still advise a high-animal-protein diet for good health and a long life!

Now you can see why the Hunza people, in defiance of all the theories of the high-protein cultists, enjoy excellent health and extraordinary longevity on the low-protein diet. Not having read the American health books which expound the virtues of a high-protein diet, they continue to eat their extremely low-protein diet (only about 1/3 of the average American's protein intake) and reap the glorious benefits in the form of total freedom from disease and a long life in youthful vitality.

According to Dr. Alexander Leaf, M.D., who visited Hunza and made an extensive study of their diet as related to their exceptionally long life, the main factors responsible for their long life are: (1) their total low-calorie diet (an average of 1900 calories a day); and (2) their predominantly vegetarian diet (only one percent of their protein intake comes from animal sources).

What can we learn from the Hunza people regarding proteins? Cut down on all proteins, especially animal proteins. The diet with the greatest potential for optimum health and a long life is a vegetarian diet with emphasis on vegetables, fruits, and seeds, nuts and grains. Homemade cottage cheese (quark) and soured milk products, which we mentioned in Chapter 3, can supplement this diet. Meat can be left out completely, or the amount consumed reduced drastically. Overindulgence in protein, especially animal protein, is incompatible with a stay-younger-longer diet. Remember: People with low-protein diets enjoy the highest life expectancy, while people who eat a high-animal-protein diet enjoy the lowest. The average life expectancy of Eskimos and Laplanders, who eat very high protein diets, is only 30-35 years.

MINERALIZED WATER—
HUNZA'S HEALTH AND LONGEVITY
SECRET NUMBER TWO

A popular nutrition columnist, Betty Lee Morales, made two visits to Hunza, and, in the course of a conversation with the Mir (the King of Hunza), asked him:

"We notice that you serve your Western guests a clear water, while you and your family drink a cloudy looking water. Please tell us the difference."

The Mir's answer reveals one of the most important health and longevity secrets from this land of superior health and perpetual youth:

"Hunza water — the kind that comes down from the glaciers—is the one we here prefer to drink. We *attribute our good health and long life to this water*, which we use both for drinking and for watering our crops. The cloudiness is caused by the minerals and trace minerals picked up as the water flows over many kinds of rocks and stones. The clear water comes from the only well in Karimibad, and, frankly, we keep it active only for our visitors; we never drink that kind ourselves," said the Mir.

"Over at the guest house we set some of this water aside in a glass. After three days, it has not settled at all. Why don't the minerals settle to the bottom?" asked Betty Lee.

"This is the secret, we believe, of the good health our water imparts," answered the Mir. "If the minerals, in microscopic particles, can't settle down in the water, perhaps they are carried into our cells and bone marrow, too. Minerals are a form of metals, I believe, and as metals they may have something to do with transference of energy. In any case, we don't need dentists, and our bones are very strong."

The erroneous belief that our bodies can use only organic minerals, and that inorganic minerals (such as those present in so-called hard, mineralized water) are not only useless, but can be harmful, has long ago been disproved. The newest worldwide research clearly shows that inorganic minerals, far from being useless or harmful, are actually essential for man's health. Both organic (as in plants and other foods) and inorganic (as in water and seawater) minerals are needed for the healthy functioning of your body. Extensive research shows that in the areas where people drink hard, mineral-rich water, there is less heart disease, diabetes, tooth decay, and hardening of the arteries. Soft water areas show the greatest incidence of the above conditions (see Chapter 3).

It has been a growing fad in recent years to drink distilled water. While drinking distilled water can be advisable in some rare cases of certain diseases (on a doctor's advice), the regular prolonged use of distilled water is definitely harmful. Man has used natural, mineral-rich waters from springs, rivers, and lakes for thousands of years and enjoyed wonderful health. Inorganic minerals in natural waters have always been an integral part of man's environment, and *an essential part of his mineral nutrition is derived from his drinking water.* To deprive yourself of this important mineral nutrition by drinking distilled water can be an extremely dangerous practice.

The Hunza example teaches us a good lesson. *Hard, highly-mineralized natural water, far from being harmful, is a very important factor in an optimum health and longevity diet.*

In this age of universal water pollution, tap water is seldom fit for drinking, and a growing number of people drink bottled water. Both natural spring water and distilled water are now sold in health food stores and supermarkets. Unless you are fortunate enough to have your own well or spring, make sure you buy the right kind of bottled water — if you wish to avoid the degenerative diseases and premature aging.

Health and Longevity Secrets from

THE ORIENT

From the East, come two of the most important health and longevity secrets: millet and sesame seeds. Health writers often speak of "miracle foods," "wonder foods," and "super foods." Millet and sesame seeds (from which halvah is made) are *true super foods*, which can help you to enjoy better health and stay younger longer.

MILLET

While millet is practically unknown in the United States and is only consumed by a small number of health-minded people (and the birds!), it is the basic grain food in most of the countries in the Middle and Far East, China, and Africa. Although it is generally believed that rice is the staple grain of the Chinese people, actually more millet than rice is consumed in China, particularly in the northern parts where the climate is too cold to grow rice. The Hindu diet is based largely on millet. It is also commonly used in large parts of Africa.

Millet is one of the most nutritious foods known to man. It is the most nutritious of the cereals, possibly sharing this distinction with buckwheat. Some anthropologists and nutritionists believe that the reason the North Chinese people are generally considered superior in physique to the South Chinese, is that the North Chinese are millet-eating people, while the South Chinese are rice-eating people.

Millet has been used by man for his food longer than any other grain. Pythagoras, over 2,500 years ago, praised the nutritional value of millet and advocated its use for his followers as the basis of their diets. Records show that the Egyptians had consumed millet for thousands of years before Pythagoras.

The nutritional value of millet is based on its following virtues:

- Millet is a high quality protein food — unique among grains, which usually are low in some essential amino acids. Buckwheat is the only other grain which contains complete protein. Amino acid composition of millet is close to that of meat or milk. Only one cup of millet cereal supplies over 20 grams (about a half day's requirement!) of high grade proteins.

- Millet is richer in vitamins and minerals than any other grains, with the exception of wild rice. According to Professors Osborne and Mendel, millet contains most of the essential vitamins and minerals and is especially rich in calcium and magnesium, as well as all the important trace elements, such as molybdenum.

- Millet is an alkaline food; again, one of the few cereal foods to be in this class. Therefore, even those who suffer from overacidity and related conditions, such as rheumatism, arthritis and diabetes, and consequently cannot use acid-forming grains such as wheat, can eat millet without any discomfort.

- Millet is a complete food in which all nutritional factors — proteins, unsaturated fatty acids, lecithin, vitamins, minerals, and carbohydrates — are balanced in ideal proportions. This explains why millet is considered to be one of the very few foods with the capacity to sustain life and good health as an exclusive item in the diet. There are many examples of famines in China, India, and Romania during which people lived almost entirely on millet for extended periods of time and remained in good health.

In addition, millet is non-fattening, which cannot be said of most other cereals. This is because millet is an alkali-forming food, and alkalies tend to dissolve and counteract the build-up of fat cells.

If you add to this the fact that millet is also one of the tastiest of all grains, then you can understand why I consider millet to be the king of all cereals, and longevity cereal number one.

How to Prepare Millet

Buy organically grown millet from your health food store. Most millet grown in the United States comes from North Dakota, where it is usually grown without the aid of sprays and chemical fertilizers (millet grows well even in comparatively poor soils).

Use only hulled millet. Do not be afraid that the hulling of millet removes its nutrients, for it does not. Millet hulls are hard outer shells, which are useless for human consumption. All proteins, vitamins, and minerals are present in hulled millet. Unhulled millet is usually sold as bird feed.

Millet, as all other grains, is best eaten cooked. Here are two ways to prepare delicious millet cereals.

MILLET CEREAL

1 cup hulled millet
3 cups water
½ cup non-instant powdered skim milk (optional)

Rinse millet in warm water and drain. Place in a pan of water mixed with powdered skim milk and heat the mixture to the boiling point. Then simmer for ten minutes, stirring occasionally to prevent sticking and burning. Remove from heat and let stand for a half hour or more. Serve with milk, honey, cold-pressed vegetable oil, or butter—or homemade applesauce. *And treat yourself to the most nutritious cereal in the world!*

MILLET CEREAL (Low-heat oven method)

Place all the ingredients, as above, in a pan with a tight cover. Use heat-proof utensil, such as pyrex, earthenware, or stainless steel. Heat the mixture to the boiling point, cover the pan, and place in an oven turned to 200° F. Leave for 3 to 4 hours, even longer if desired, but the cereal will be ready to eat in about three hours.

This is a superior method of preparing millet cereal because of the low temperature, which makes the nutrients of millet, particularly the proteins, more assimilable. Serve in the same manner as described in the first recipe.

SESAME SEEDS

While millet has been used by man longer than any other grain, sesame seeds have been used longer than any other seed, going back to the earliest stages of civilization. Cultivated for thousands of years, sesame is named in many ancient writings as a special longevity food. It is used widely in Africa and in the Middle and

Far East. In India and China, sesame is a staple food. Armenian Turks use it in a liquid form called *Matahini*, which is considered to be a respected rejuvenator of mental and physical capacities and endurance. In Israel, Turkey, and Arabian countries, a candy made from sesame seeds — halvah — is very popular. The women of ancient Babylonia used halvah to enhance their sex appeal and to restore the virility of their men.

Halvah is available even in the United States, mostly from ethnic markets and delicatessens, and also from health food stores. Health food stores also sell a butter-like spread made from sesame seeds, called *Tahini.*

While millet is the King of Cereals, sesame is the King of Seeds. Sesame seeds are extremely nutritious. They are richer in calcium than milk, cheese, or nuts. Their protein content is 19 percent to 28 percent higher than that of meat, and sesame protein is of very high value, comparable in quality to the protein in meat. Sesame seeds are especially good sources of the important amino acid methionine, which is otherwise scarce in proteins of plant sources.

Sesame seeds are also very rich in unsaturated fatty acids — up to 50 percent of the seed is oil. They are also rich in vitamin E and B vitamins: niacin, inositol and choline.

Both millet and sesame, by the way, are excellent sources of lecithin, an organic phosphorized fat which is a chief constituent of brain and nerve tissues, and an essential component of semen. Lecithin is an effective aid in keeping your blood vessels free from cholesterol deposits. It is also vitally important for the proper function of endocrine glands which are to a great extent responsible for your looking and feeling young: pituitary, pineal and sex glands.

Sesame seeds, in combination with honey (halvah), can be considered an important sexual virility food.

French doctors who investigated the popular belief that halvah is a powerful aphrodisiac, found that the rejuvenative property of halvah can be scientifically explained. Sesame seeds have abundant magnesium and potassium, and honey is rich in aspartic acid, one of the amino acids. Some doctors have used a very similar prescription formula — the potassium and magnesium salts of aspartic acid—to treat women with "the housewife syndrome," or chronic fatigue, insomnia, and lethargy in lovemaking—87 percent responded with a startling improvement in condition. Aspartic acid is an important rejuvenative factor, particularly for sexual rejuvenation.

Sesame seeds are sold in most health food stores. Use only raw, unroasted, *hulled* sesame seeds. Make sure the seeds you buy were hulled mechanically, without the use of chemicals. To my knowledge, there is at least one company that produces such sesame seeds: International Protein Industries, Inc., P.O. Box 871, Smithtown, N.Y. 11787.

Sesame seeds can be used in many ways to enhance your diet. Sprinkle them on cereals or salads, mix or blend them in drinks, use in soups or dips, or make your own homemade halvah.

Here is the recipe for it:

HALVAH*

1 cup sesame seeds
2 tsp. coagulated, natural honey

Grind sesame seeds in an electric seed grinder. Pour sesame meal into a large cup and knead honey into it with a large spoon until honey is well mixed in and halvah acquires the consistency of hard dough. Serve it as it is, or make small balls and roll in whole sesame seeds, freshly shredded coconut, sunflower seeds, or fresh wheat germ — and enjoy one of the finest and best-tasting health and virility foods in the world!

The Romans had an old custom of giving soldiers an emergency ration — cakes made of sesame seeds and honey. Experience had convinced them that men could walk farther and survive longer on this ration than on any other food of equal weight.

To assure freshness, keep sesame seeds and halvah refrigerated.

---

*) Note: Commercial halvah is made with sugar and egg white, which is used as a binding agent. I have formulated this simple recipe using only sesame seeds and honey. It holds together well, especially if sesame seeds are ground very fine and if hard, coagulated honey is used. And it's simply super-delicious! Make sure, however, that the sesame seeds are 100 percent fresh, not rancid. They turn stale and rancid in about 6 months after they are harvested.

10

Health and Longevity Secrets from

MEXICO

Mexico is one of the countries in which I have had the opportunity to travel and study extensively. In the 60's and 70's I directed a biological medical clinic in Mexico, where I had an opportunity to observe the results of many rejuvenative therapies employed at the clinic.

Herbal healing science is highly advanced in Mexico. It has ancient traditions, stemming from the extensive use of herbs for healing and revitalization by Mayan, Aztecs, and other native Indians. While the popularity of herbal medicines has declined during this century in the rest of the world, in Mexico herbs are used almost as much now as they ever were. Every market place features many *yerbalistas*, who are well educated in the medicinal properties of Mexican native herbs. I dare say that even today more people in Mexico use medicinal herbs for healing than chemical drugs from *farmacias*.

By living in Mexico for many years, I also discovered that the traditional Mexican diet features several powerful health and longevity factors. Let's look at these first.

PAPAYA, LIME, AND CHILI

The Mexican contribution to my international list of health-building longevity foods are three foods which are used by the Mexicans as staples in their traditional diet: papaya, lime, and chili.

Papaya is a tropical fruit which grows abundantly in Mexico. It is rich in the enzyme *papain*, which is an effective digestive aid. Papain helps break down protein into amino acids and makes them easily assimilable. Papaya is also extremely rich in vitamins — particularly vitamin C — and minerals.

Mexicans eat papaya as a dessert, especially after a protein-rich meal. This is an excellent habit, since it can truthfully be said that *we are not what we eat*, but *what we assimilate*. Papaya helps the digestive tract to digest and assimilate protein-rich foods more effectively.

Papaya is also an excellent cleansing food, with many remarkable therapeutic properties. In our clinic we used papaya and papaya juice to treat many conditions, including digestive disorders, arthritis, obesity, and kidney diseases, with remarkable results.

Papayas are now sold in most supermarkets in the United States. They are usually imported from Mexico or Hawaii. Health food stores also sell papaya juice, papaya pulp, and digestive tablets containing papain.

Limes are another digestion-promoting food that Mexicans use liberally. In fact, in the traditional Mexican diet, limes are used with every conceivable food or drink: Mexicans serve cut limes with all orders in restaurants; they squeeze lime on all fruits and vegetables, including papaya; they squeeze it into juices and drinks, including beer and tequila; and they squeeze lime juice on meat, fish, and any other kind of prepared dish. Limes are also considered to be one of the best medicines, especially for colds, skin diseases, stomach disorders, dysentery ("turista") or for disinfection and healing of fresh wounds and scratches. Even for mosquito bites!

The medicinal value of the lime is well documented by extensive research. It is a powerful antiseptic. It is also antiscorbutic: that is, it will help to prevent disease and will assist in cleansing the system of impurities. Lime or lemon juice is also a wonderful stimulant to the liver; it dissolves uric acid crystals in the tissues; and it is an excellent help in the digestion of food. It is rich in digestive enzymes and its acid property helps to create an acid condition in the stomach, which is necessary for protein and mineral digestion. Lemon and lime juice are specific in the treatment of such conditions as asthma, colds, liver complaints, scurvy, dysentery, fevers, and digestive problems.

In recent years, the addition of apple cider vinegar to the diet has become very popular in the United States. As people grow older, their digestion tends to become sluggish, mostly because of the diminished secretion of hydrochloric acid in the stomach. Apple cider vinegar, although it does not substitute for the hydrochloric acid entirely, creates an acid condition in the stomach and helps to improve digestion, especially of proteins and minerals. In Mexico, lime juice is used for the same purpose. In my experience, lime or lemon juice in small amounts is preferable to apple cider vinegar, as it has, in addition to its beneficial acids, many important vitamins, minerals, and enzymes.

Finally, *chili* is another Mexican contribution to better health and longer life. Nowhere in the world is chili consumed to the extent that it is in Mexico. As with lime juice, chili powder is sprinkled on virtually everything, including oranges, apples, mangoes, and watermelon. It is also added to practically every cooked food, and not in just microscopic amounts to spike or enhance the natural flavors in food, but in such huge amounts that most non-Mexicans have to gasp for air and water after a single bite of any traditional Mexican food.

Mexicans use many kinds of chilies, some mild, like our regular green or red peppers, some so strong that a mere rub on the skin will produce a blister. The strong, tiny chili peppers are used mostly for cooking and making salza, a Mexican dressing prepared with chili, tomatoes, garlic, and onions. Milder chilies are often eaten raw in salads. Cayenne, or red pepper, is the most commonly used chili throughout Mexico.

Can these strong peppers be healthful? While mustard and white and black pepper, which are commonly used in the United States, are definitely harmful, toxic, and irritating to the delicate linings of the stomach and bowels, cayenne pepper or chili is extremely beneficial and soothing. It has many wonderful medicinal properties. It stimulates circulation, it helps digestion by stimulating the production of enzymes and hydrochloric acid in the stomach, it exerts a beneficial, stimulating action on kidneys, spleen, and pancreas, and it is considered to be a powerful general tonic and stimulant. If you ask an average Mexican why he is so healthy, he will inevitably answer: "chili."

By the way, chilies are extremely rich in vitamins, minerals, and enzymes, especially in vitamin C.

My conclusion is that chili has definite health-promoting and age-retarding properties if used in moderate amounts.

MEXICAN REJUVENATIVE HERBS

Herbs are used in every country and by every race for healing and rejuvenating purposes, and have been so used throughout the ages. Mexico has many potent herbs that are used for healing disease. Since this book deals primarily with secrets of staying young and living long, two special herbs come to my mind: damiana and sarsaparilla.

Damiana is mostly known and highly regarded as an aphrodisiac. It is used widely, not only in Mexico, but in most Central and South American countries. It is sold by every Mexican village or town herbalist.

There are many kinds of damiana. The kind mostly used in Mexico is known botanically as *Turnera aphrodisiaca*. It grows in Baja California, all over Mexico, and in Central and South America. Damiana grown in Baja California is considered to be the most potent. Damiana grows as a shrub or small tree, with small narrow leaves. The leaves are dried and used mostly as tea, which has a slightly bitter taste.

Damiana is an old remedy for sexual impotence. It strengthens and enhances the function of male reproductive organs. Damiana is also known to be a tonic for the nerves and is used in cases of mental and physical exhaustion. In addition, it is a stimulant to the kidneys and increases the flow of urine. Damiana is prepared like most herb teas: 1 tsp. of dried leaves to 1 cup of water. Pour boiling water over the leaves and let stand and steep for 15 minutes. Take one cup twice a day. Most health food stores and herb stores in the United States sell damiana.

Sarsaparilla is another Mexican rejuvenative herb. Sarsaparilla is a tropical plant which grows mostly in Honduras, Mexico, Jamaica, and Ecuador, but also in China and Japan. The botanical name is *Smilax Medica* or *Smilax Regalii*. It is an evergreen herb, and the root is the only part used for medicinal purposes.

Sarsaparilla is considered to be a powerful blood purifier and also is used for such conditions as chronic rheumatism, skin disorders, psoriasis, general weakness, and sexual impotence. It is considered to be a potent antidote for the toxic effects of any strong poison.

But, for the purpose of this presentation, the most important fact about sarsaparilla is that it is a natural source of male and female sex hormones, which are involved in keeping the body and mind young. American and Mexican scientists discovered — independently of each other — that sarsaparilla roots contain *testosterone*, a male sex hormone. And recently it was discovered that sarsaparilla also contains *progesterone*, a female sex hormone. Even *cortin* — one of the adrenal hormones —was found in sarsaparilla.

In recent times, therefore, Mexican and South American pharmaceutical companies have been manufacturing male and female sex hormone tablets from natural hormones isolated from sarsaparilla.

It is generally considered that the strength of the endocrine glands, and particularly the sex glands, and their ability to produce sufficient hormones, is directly related to the general vitality and healthy functioning of the body. Sexual virility largely determines man's youthfulness, health, vitality, and longevity. Likewise, plentiful sex hormone production in the female makes her look, feel, and act young. The decline in sex hormone production results in gradual aging and decreased life span. Therefore, sarsaparilla can be listed as one of the most important natural longevity herbs. It can help to supply the missing hormones and bring the spark of youth back into your life.

Sarsaparilla roots (the red Honduras sarsaparilla is considered the most potent) are boiled in water for 15 to 30 minutes, and the decoction is drunk as a tea twice a day. Use one ounce of the root to one pint of water.

Speaking of herbs, perhaps this will be the proper place for a few other herbal secrets, especially for female rejuvenation. The aging processes in the female are accelerated after menopause, when the glandular

DR. PAAVO AIROLA

activity slows down and sex hormone deficiencies, especially the deficiency of estrogen, will manifest itself. Many women drug themselves with the synthetic hormone, estrogen, to slow down the aging processes. This can be very dangerous, as it is well known that taking synthetic estrogen can lead to the development of cancer. In addition to sarsaparilla there are several other herbal sources of natural estrogen, which is totally harmless: licorice, false unicorn roots, black cohosh, and elder flowers.

Herbs should be used as herb teas. Take 1 tsp. of dried herbs (individual or mixed) per cup of water. Place herbs in boiling water, remove pot from the heat, and steep for 15-20 minutes. Strain. Drink one cup two times a day. If herbs are available only in capsule or tablet form, don't swallow them as such, but crush the tablets and empty the capsules into the boiling water and use them for making a herb tea.

11

Health and Longevity Secrets from

CHINA

Since the communist take-over several decades ago, China has been out of contact with the rest of the world. The bamboo curtain is now open, and many Western travelers are anxiously looking East in hopes of learning something from this, perhaps, the oldest civilization in the world.

Already we are astounded at some of the medical secrets that are coming out of China. Acupuncture is one of them. This 5,000-year-old Chinese art of healing has amazed the entire Western medical world. "It may well be ... that the latter half of the 20th Century will one day be called the Golden Age of Acupuncture," wrote the *New York Times*. Western doctors have learned that the Chinese technique of inserting needles at various points in the body can have dramatic curative effects on a wide range of ailments extending from headaches and muscular pains to serious heart disease, arthritis, diabetes and other disorders.

But even while China was securely behind the bamboo curtain, longevity-conscious Westerners had continuous contact with the East through the use of famous oriental herbs — notably ginseng, and gotu kola. These two herbs, used in China and its close neighbors, Manchuria and Korea, for thousands of years, are credited with remarkable youth-promoting and age-retarding properties.

GINSENG

Ginseng (Panax ginseng) is the most famous and the most potent energizing and rejuvenating plant. The roots of the ginseng bear a remarkable resemblance to the shape and form of man. This is why the Chinese called the plant, *ginseng*, or "man-plant."

Ginseng has been used by 500 million Chinese and many more millions of other Orientals for over 5,000 years as an effective aphrodisiac, rejuvenator, revitalizer, and cure-all for a variety of ills. Ginseng is now used widely even in the United States. In spite of the fact that ginseng is very expensive in China — valued almost at the price of gold — it is bought and used by millions of people. In some cases, the very poor people sell their last possessions to buy this herb with the alleged miraculous properties.

Is the reputation of ginseng based on ignorance and superstition, or can it be substantiated by scientific research?

Several studies of ginseng's alleged properties have been conducted in various research centers around the world. So far, it has been found that substances in ginseng increase mental efficiency, enhance resistance to stress and infections, improve general metabolism, reduce cholesterol accumulation in arteries, improve circulation, increase endocrine activity, purify blood, reduce fatigue, and protect against radiation.

The Russian Institute of Experimental Medicine made an extensive study of ginseng and its claimed medicinal and rejuvenating properties. They discovered that ginseng grows only in radioactive soil, and that the roots of the plant itself contain many radioactive properties. In fact, this radioactive property of ginseng helps the collectors of the wild ginseng to locate the plant. The ginseng plant emits its radioactive rays, which are evidenced by a distinct glow at night. Ginseng hunters go out during the night and shoot colored arrows at the glowing plants. The next day, they locate the plants marked by the arrows and dig the roots.

Russian researchers also have found that the claims the Orientals were making about ginseng were true: it strengthens the heart, revitalizes the nervous system, increases hormone production, and stimulates cell growth and activity. After the results of this research were reported to the Russian Government, it immediately ordered the establishment of huge plantations of ginseng in Southern Siberia. The Siberian variety of ginseng is known as *Eleutherococcus senticosus*. Russians also buy most of the ginseng produced in North Korea, while most of the ginseng produced in South Korea is sold to the United States.

Ginseng (*Panax quinquefolius*) grows wild in some parts of central United States. There are also many plantations, both here and in other parts of the world, where ginseng is grown commercially. The plant must be at least 6 years old before the roots can be collected.

The bulk of all ginseng sold in the United States comes from Korea and China. Ginseng is sold in all health food stores in powder, tablet, or capsule form. It is also available as a whole root or packaged in tea bags.

HYDROCOTYLE ASIATICA MINOR (GOTU KOLA)

Hydrocotyle Asiatica Minor is another well-known rejuvenator. It is a small plant that grows only in certain jungle districts of the Oriental tropics.

It was popularized by the renowned Chinese scholar and herbalist, Professor Li Chung Yun, who lived to be 256 years of age. Don't laugh! Professor Li Chung Yun's age is well documented. Being a world-famous scholar, he was in the public eye for over 200 years. At the age of 100, he was awarded by the Chinese government a special Honor Citation for extraordinary services to his country. This document is available in existing archives. For over 150 years after the award, the Professor was visited by countless Western scholars and students. It is reported that he gave a series of 28 lectures at the University of Sinkiang when he was over 200 years old.

Being born in 1677 and having died in 1933, his life spanned four centuries — 17th, 18th, 19th, and 20th. He enjoyed excellent health, outlived 23 wives (he was living with his 24th wife at the time of his death), and kept his own natural teeth and hair. Those who saw him at the age of 200 testified that he did not appear much older than a man in his fifties. Professor Li Chung Yun attributed his longevity to his lifelong vegetarian diet and the regular use of the age-retarding herbs, ginseng and gotu kola; plus — may I add, an important plus —to his "inward calm." He used gotu kola and ginseng daily in the form of tea.

British, French, and Ceylonese researchers, who made studies and clinical tests on Hydrocotyle Asiatica Minor, agree that the plant contains an unknown vitamin, which they termed "vitamin X," or the "youth vitamin." This new vitamin, they say, has a rejuvenating effect on the brain cells and on the endocrine glands. The French government was so impressed by the research on the rejuvenative properties of this plant that it established several large plantations and experimental research stations in Algeria.

Hydrocotyle Asiatica Minor is available in health food stores, both in pure form, as Gotu Kola, or as an ingredient in an herbal blend called Fo-ti-tieng.

The effectiveness of these Oriental rejuvenation herbs is attributed to the fact that they have a stimulating effect on all vital body functions by keeping endocrine and sex glands in peak working condition far into advanced age, and by increasing the production of life-giving hormones, which are the actual "Fountains of Youth." They also exert an energizing effect on nerve and brain functions and keep blood free from age-causing toxins. Well, if they can do only a fraction of all this they can rightfully be called the "Herbal Fountains of Youth."

Note: There has been some confusion regarding *Fo-ti-tieng.* Some writers claim that Fo-ti-tieng is an herb (as did even this writer earlier, misled by unreliable sources of information). Actually, Fo-ti-tieng is a trade name for an herbal formula made from three different herbs, one of which is *Hydrocotyle Asiatica Minor.*

12

Health and Longevity Secrets from

PITCAIRN ISLAND

"From where?" I hear your perplexed question. Even the veteran health book readers, for whom Hunza is a household word, have, in all probability, never heard of Pitcairn Island.

Pitcairn Island is located in the South Pacific, just below the Tropic of Capricorn, south-east of Tahiti. In 1789, the mutineers of the legendary pirated British armed transport, *Bounty*, led by Fletcher Christian, established an utopian commune on this remote Pacific island, which has been recently stirring much interest among the modern longevity and health researchers. Although the total population of Pitcairn Island has never reached over 233 (and now, mostly due to emigration, has dwindled to 73), the island has lured several investigators and scientists who were impressed by the exceptional health and longevity of these seventh-generation descendants of nine British navymen and their brown Tahitian concubines.

American physician, Dr. David Gibson, of Grand Prairie, who visited Pitcairn Island recently and made a thorough examination and study of their health condition says, "It would be difficult to find a comparable population anywhere in the world as healthy, robust, and physically fit as these people." He found that "apart from some minor surgical procedures, there really isn't much to do" there. Although life expectancy studies have never been made on the Pitcairners, most observers have found that the average age of death is in the mid or late seventies — this in spite of the unusual hazards posed in daily life on the island, and that one in every five Pitcairners die by accident at sea, in falls from cliffs, or in hunting mishaps.

Ian Ball, U.S. correspondent for the *Daily Telegraph* of London, and the author of the immensely interesting book, *Pitcairn: Children of Mutiny* (Little, Brown and Company, 380 pp.), has spent much time on Pitcairn Island and has made a thorough study of the history, the living and eating habits, and the health condition of the people there. He writes ". . . without question (they) are the most physically robust society I have ever encountered."

Dr. Gibson was amazed at the youthful vigor and stamina demonstrated by the "old" Pitcairners. Men well over seventy scramble up rope ladders to the decks of ships like only twenty-year-olds elsewhere might do.

When these and other researchers try to pinpoint the actual causes of the exceptional health and longevity of the Pitcairners, they invariably list their diet as the most important cause. Partly as a result of the tight isolation from the "civilized" world, partly because of the limited availability of foods, but mainly as a result of the dietary laws of their religion, these human relics of the *Bounty* saga live on a diet which enlightened modern nutritionists have found to be the ideal program for optimum health and long life. At the end of the last century, *all* Pitcairners were converted to the Seventh-Day Adventist faith. Consequently, they are basically vegetarians, the staples of their diet being the abundance of delicious fruits, berries, and vegetables that grow on their island. They do eat some fish, following the injunction in Leviticus to eat only "whatsoever hath fins and scales in the waters," avoiding completely cray fish and shell fish, which abound in Pitcairn waters.

Needless to say, they do not drink or smoke, and most do not use tea or coffee. Homemade fruit drinks and juices are their staple drinks — pineapple juice, wild strawberry juice, orange juice, etc. Dairy products and milk are almost non-existent. All attempts to introduce dairy farming to the island have failed — the cows kept falling off the cliffs. With the exception of imported canned butter, the islanders use hardly any dairy products.

PITCAIRNERS' HEALTH AND LONGEVITY SECRET NUMBER ONE

As I studied the various living and eating habits of the Pitcairners, trying to pinpoint the prime cause of their superior health and vitality and exceptional longevity, I uncovered one factor, which I learned from my teacher, Are Waerland, 30 years ago, but which has been somewhat forgotten in this, the start-the-day-with-a-hearty-protein-breakfast era. Pitcairners eat their breakfast at noon! Although they start their day at sunrise, or about 5 A.M., and do all kinds of heavy physical labor and activity all morning, they do not eat any solid protein foods until a late breakfast at midday. They start their day with a large mug of pure well water, and then snack on fresh fruits or fruit juices now and then as the morning passes. This practice is of tremendous importance for their health and vitality, as you will soon see.

It is appalling how many of our nutrition advisors recommend eating a large protein-rich breakfast as soon as you get out of bed in the morning. This is contrary to all scientific and empirical evidence that I could uncover during more than 40 years of nutrition research.

During the night, from about 11 P.M. to 5 A.M., your digestive, assimilative, and restorative systems are busy at work, while your eliminative system is at rest. The morning hours from about 5 A.M. to 11 A.M., constitute a period of cleansing and elimination, when the blood-stream is heavily charged with the waste products of metabolism carried out during the night, and the eliminative organs are doing their job of cleansing the system of impurities and toxins — through the skin, through the lungs, and through the kidneys and alimentary canal. "Morning breath" is just one indication of such elimination. Lack of appetite in the early morning is another. Eating a large breakfast as soon as you get up will disrupt this cleansing process and interrupt the elimination. What your body needs in the early morning is plenty of fresh air, lots of liquids, fresh juicy fruits, and vigorous physical work or exercise to help your body complete its cleansing and eliminating process. Then, but not before, you are ready for breakfast.

Paul Bragg, a veteran health-builder and life-extension expert, had a good way of putting it. He said, "you must earn your breakfast." So, he goes for a long walk, swims, or does heavy exercise in the morning before he is ready for food. This is how it should be. This is how *all* "natural" people—the natives known for their excellent health—always do. They get up early in the morning, normally "with the sun," and immediately go to their heavy chores: feeding the animals or taking them to the pasture, milking the cows, working in the garden or fields, fishing or hunting — or whatever their particular work or lifestyle is. For women it is usually work around the house, preparing the breakfast, baking bread, cleaning the house, etc., etc. Then—*several hours later* — after hard work and plenty of perspiration, they are ready for breakfast. This routine is followed by all healthy natives everywhere: in Hunza, in Bulgaria, in Russia, in Scandinavia, by North, Central, and South American Indians, *as well as by Pitcairners*.

To eat a large protein-rich breakfast right after you've gotten out of bed and when you really are not hungry, is to do yourself a great disservice. This routine is a sure road to premature aging, impaired health, disease, and short life.

Yet, this is exactly what most of our misinformed "authorities" advise us to do. You may not believe this, but I have heard it with my own ears. After a lecture given by one of those hearty-protein-breakfast advocates, a rather obese lady said to the lecturer, "But, I don't feel hungry in the morning!" To which the lecturer replied: "Don't wait until you get hungry. Eat a large breakfast of liver, steak, eggs, and milk, and you won't get hungry during your working hours."

"Breakfast like a king, lunch like a queen, and dine like a pauper" is a false precept, contrived by our misled and confused nutritionists. You will be better off if you "Breakfast like a pauper, lunch like a king, and dine like a queen." There are all kinds of *theories* regarding eating and drinking — *when* you should or shouldn't eat or drink — *theories invented by scientists*. To answer the question for yourself *when you* should eat or drink, you don't need scientists or their theories. *Nature* has provided a built-in mechanism within your brain which will tell you unmistakably when you should eat or drink. *You should eat when you are hungry, and drink when you are thirsty.* Contrarywise, you should *never drink when you are not thirsty, nor eat when you are not hungry.* Most people are not hungry at five or six in the morning when they just get out of bed, and before they leave for work. To eat a huge protein-rich breakfast at such a time is to work against your body's own timetable and its requirements. This can seriously endanger your health.

Follow the example of the Pitcairners—drink water, diluted fruit juice, or herb tea the first thing in the morning; then an hour or two later, snack on fresh, juicy fruit, and eat a hearty breakfast at 11:00 or noon —and see what a difference it will make in the way you feel! To achieve optimum health and long life, you have to work with nature—and its own timetable—not against it.

Note: The above-mentioned advice applies to adults only. Children do need to eat in the morning as their metabolism and cleansing processes are different; children of school age especially should have breakfast before leaving for school.

13

Health and Longevity Secrets from

AMERICA

As could be expected, the American contribution to the health and longevity secrets comes in pill form — vitamins, minerals, and food supplements. Since we are more youth-oriented than any other people, a great deal of our attention has been directed not so much towards finding the ways of improving health and preventing the aging processes, as to preserving the appearance of youth. Since Americans are also extraordinarily drug-or pill-oriented, our "youth researchers" and "youth doctors" are trying to find the secret of youth in a single vitamin or other food substance; a fountain of youth in a glass of miracle juice, or a little tablet or gelatin capsule that will perform the wonder of rejuvenation.

Although, as I said in the Introduction, the true secrets of staying young and living long involve the total approach and dedicated effort in many areas, such as nutrition, lifestyle, exercise, peace of mind, mental and spiritual attitudes, etc., I am happy to report that there are some specific isolated vitamins, minerals, trace elements, and other food substances that do indeed possess unique rejuvenative properties and can help prevent the aging processes, or even reverse them. One of the researchers who was interested in the prospect of prolongation of life, Dr. Paul de Kruif, says that

WORLDWIDE SECRETS FOR STAYING YOUNG

vitamins are "potent chemicals that will help stretch out your span of productive vitality. We now know that the time to try to push back senility is before we're old in years." Stressing that nutritional deficiencies may be the main cause of premature aging, he continues, "What we eat—while seemingly quite adequate—may mean the premature aging of many of us. But by using chemical knowledge now available, this premature aging can be reversed." Many other researchers feel that in the "chemical knowledge," or in the nutritive chemicals—vitamins, minerals, etc.—may be hidden the true secret of extended youth.

Let's look at some of these.

VITAMIN E

Of all the vitamins, vitamin E is the anti-aging vitamin number one. This vitamin has been credited with being a miracle youth, virility, and vitality vitamin — a vitamin which can reverse the aging processes and keep you younger longer.

One of the leading American experts on aging — its causes, prevention, and cure—is Dr. Aloys L. Tappel, a biochemist at the University of California, and professor of Food Science and Technology at Davis College. Dr. Tappel says, "Aging is due to the process of oxidation." He writes:

"Aging of our bodies appears to be influenced by an intracellular tug of war going on between two factors acting upon a third: intensity and duration of radiation-like effects, polyunsaturated lipids upon which they act, and the vitamin E available to protect them from excessive destruction."

Dr. Tappel says that as we become older, the oxygenation of our cells is diminished, and because of increased oxidation, certain substances, called *free-radicals*, are formed within our cells. These free-radicals have a destructive effect on normal cell metabolism, causing damage and contributing to the aging processes. "Perhaps the reason some people look older than their years is that they have been more vulnerable to this damage than those who don't show their age," says Dr. Tappel.

As I explained in Chapter 1, free-radicals are results of lipid (fat) peroxidation. Free-radicals not only cause cancer and contribute to the development of other degenerative diseases, but they directly contribute to premature aging by causing so-called cross-linkage in connective tissues of the body—collagen, elastin, and reticulin. This causes wrinkled and leathery skin, stiff and immobile joints, hardening of arteries, and other impairment in many vital body functions.

Dr. Tappel's prescription for preventing development of free-radicals and, consequently, premature aging is vitamin E. Vitamin E is one of the most powerful natural antioxidants and free-radical deactivators. Dr. Tappel says: "in normal humans, vitamin E, contained in unsaturated vegetable fat, acts to prevent the formation of free-radicals and serves as a built-in protection against accelerated aging."

By the way, vitamin E deficiency also causes the formation of age-pigments, ceroid and lipofuscin, which are thought to contribute to premature aging.

Since our typical American diet is grossly deficient in vitamin E, supplementing it with extra vitamin E in capsule form would be one of the best things you could do for yourself to prevent premature aging, extend life, and stay younger longer.

The best natural sources of vitamin E are whole grains, seeds, and nuts, and some unrefined, cold-pressed vegetable oils. Refined foods, such as white flour or bread, or processed oils, do not contain enough vitamin E to keep you young, because most of the vitamin E in them has been removed or destroyed in processing.

Vitamin E in capsule form is sold in all health food stores and drug stores. Most doctors recommend doses up to 600 IU as perfectly safe. Older people can take twice as much. Those who suffer from serious diseases, especially high blood pressure, overactive thyroid, or heart damage from rheumatic fever, should not take high dosages of vitamin E, and should consult their doctors regarding the proper dosage.

Another noted scientist who believes that vitamin E can help to control or even reverse the aging processes is Dr. Hans Selye, of the University of Montreal. Dr. Selye is the author of the famous stress theory: that all diseases, including premature aging, are caused by stresses which the weakened body is unable to counteract. Vitamin E is one of our basic anti-stress vitamins. It increases the body's resistance to stresses by improving circulation, strengthening the heart, preventing oxidation, and increasing the oxygenation of all tissues and cells. Dr. Selye tells how in animal studies he was able to cause all signs and symptoms of "old age" by deliberately withholding vitamin E from the test animals. Conversely, in the other group of test animals, life and youth was prolonged through the use of vitamin E.

In addition to all the health-improving and age-retarding properties of vitamin E mentioned so far, it is an effective natural antioxidant that can work on the cellular level, preventing lipid peroxidation within the microsomes and mitochondria. Vitamin E also combats many forms of environmental pollution and has a beneficial stimulating effect on the endocrine glandular system.

As you can see, vitamin E is one of the truly miraculous, health-building, and health-restoring substances. It helps to save lives by favorably influencing such conditions as heart disease, diabetes, arthritis, arteriosclerosis, varicose veins, ulcers, etc. Vitamin E is also a potent rejuvenator of male and female fertility and virility. It has a strong regenerative and stimulating effect on all sexual and reproductive functions. It can help prevent miscarriages and spontaneous abortions; it increases fertility of both the male and female; it can restore virility in impotent men and banish frigidity in women. Although you may have heard repeatedly the official medical line that "there is absolutely no evidence" that vitamin E is a sex rejuvenator, there are dozens of reliable clinical studies from around the world which show that vitamin E, indeed, can do all of the things mentioned above. By improving and regenerating the functions of your sex glands, vitamin E can definitely help you to stay younger longer.

It is obvious from the above evidence that vitamin E should be included in your optimum health and longevity program.

VITAMIN C

As I stressed in Chapter 1, many scientists believe that one of the basic causes of premature aging is the degenerative processes in collagen and elastin, the intercellular cements which hold the cells together. This deterioration in collagen is largely caused by a vitamin C deficiency. Physiological changes in collagen, caused by a deficiency of vitamin E, peroxidation, and free-radicals, lead to such symptoms as wrinkles, flabbiness, and skin discolorations, in addition to adversely affecting all the metabolic processes in the body, and speeding up the aging process.

This has been clearly shown by Dr. W.J. McCormick's work. Also, Dr. Tappel stresses that in addition to vitamin E, vitamin C can help to retard the aging processes by improving and strengthening the cellular and collagen integrity. Dr. Tapple recommends supplementing the diet with large doses of vitamin C.

A Japanese researcher, Dr. M. Higuchi, recently reported that his studies show a definite relationship between vitamin C levels in the diet and hormone production of the sex glands. He says that older people, particularly, need larger amounts of vitamin C to assure adequate sex hormone production.

Vitamin C is vitally involved in all the functions of your body. It is our most potent anti-toxin. It helps your body to protect itself against every stress and every condition threatening your health. Since aging processes are often associated with various conditions of diminished health, vitamin C becomes an important life-prolongator. By improving cell breathing, vitamin C prevents the premature aging of cells. It also has a beneficial stimulating effect on adrenal glands, helping them in hormone production, particularly in production of cortisone. "You are as young as your glands," believe many scientists. Vitamin C helps your glands to work at the peak of their capacity and keep you younger longer.

A stay-younger-longer program should include large doses of vitamin C — 3,000 to 5,000 mg. a day for adults.

VITAMIN A

It has been established by research that the oxygenation of the tissues is enhanced by a combination of vitamins E and A. Vitamin A increases the permeability of blood capillaries. The capillaries carry oxygen and other nutritive substances to every cell of your body. The more permeable these capillary walls, the more oxygen can be delivered to the cells. Thus, vitamin A is a third vitamin (in addition to E and C) that can improve cell oxygenation; and efficient cell oxygenation is the ultimate secret of perpetual youth.

Vitamin A helps keep your skin youthful at any age, by preventing drying of the skin and keeping it free from blemishes.

Vitamin A is also a powerful antioxidant and free-radical deactivator. In addition, it helps decrease serum cholesterol.

Two scientists from Columbia University, Drs. H.C. Sherman and Oswald A. Roels, demonstrated that vitamin A helps to prevent premature aging and increases life expectancy by as much as 10 to 20 percent. It regulates the stability of tissue in cell walls — cell membranes break down when there is a lack of vitamin A. Vitamin A is also essential for the health of all mucous linings and membranes in the body.

The best natural sources of vitamin A are carrots, tomatoes, and green leafy vegetables. Fish liver oils are the richest natural source. Vitamin A capsules are sold in all health food stores. Optimal preventive doses are 25,000 to 30,000 U.S.P. units a day. Excessively large doses of vitamin A can be toxic when taken for prolonged periods of time. It would be wise, therefore, to make 2-3 week intervals every few months if you take doses larger than 30,000.

Note: If you suffer from any serious illness, or are doubtful about the proper dosage of vitamins and supplements, have a nutritionally oriented doctor prescribe the most suitable dosage *for you.*

B-COMPLEX VITAMINS

Although in this book I mention only a few vitamins, minerals, and other supplements which have been scientifically proven to have age-preventing and life-prolonging properties, I am sure you understand that *all* vitamins, minerals and trace elements are important in the overall program of keeping healthy and staying young.

From the B-vitamin complex, which includes over twenty different vitamins, specific vitamins that are involved in keeping you young are:

• *Pantothenic acid (vitamin B₅)* is of specific importance to women who wish to delay the onset of menopause. Animal studies show, however, that pantothenic acid can delay the onset of old age both for men and women. Dr. Roger J. Williams, who discovered this vitamin, demonstrated in his animal studies at the University of Texas that it increased the life span of both male and female mice by about 20 percent.

Pantothenic acid, as Dr. Williams found, is the active ingredient in royal jelly, long known for its remarkable life-extending properties.

Pantothenic acid is a powerful anti-stress vitamin. It is a constituent of co-enzyme A, which is involved in energy metabolism. It is essential for the production of adrenal hormones, especially cortisone, which can protect against every form of stress. Pantothenic acid helps fight infections and speeds recovery from ill health. It is vital for the normal development and function of the central nervous system. It has been reported that gray hair returned to its original color when pantothenic acid was taken together with other B vitamins, especially PABA, biotin, and folic acid.

• *Thiamine (vitamin B₁)* is called the anti aging vitamin. It is essential for effective protein metabolism. It promotes cellular growth, protects the heart muscle, stimulates brain action, and is vital for the health of the entire nervous system. It helps prevent premature aging by improving circulation, increasing stamina, and stimulating the pituitary gland to keep sexual desires normal. The main value of thiamine as an anti-aging vitamin is that it regulates and normalizes oxidative metabolism by means of its function of transforming glucose to energy — thus, it protects against oxidation.

• *Riboflavin (vitamin B₂)* helps to keep the youthful appearance of your skin, nails, and hair. It also helps to prevent premature wrinkling of the facial skin, as well as the skin on the arms. Prolonged deficiency of B_2 can result in "whistle marks" — wrinkles around the mouth — which are usually associated with premature aging processes in women.

• *Niacin (vitamin B₃).* According to the famous Canadian researcher, Dr. Abram Hoffer, the world's leading authority on the therapeutic uses of niacin, an optimum diet, supplemented with adequate amounts of all vitamins and minerals, plus mega-doses of niacin, will extend life by 10 to 20 years. He recommends 3,000 mg. of niacin (niacinamide) a day as a regular dose for old, senile people. Dr. Hoffer says that heart attacks, strokes, and physical and mental senility can be prevented by large doses of niacin.

Niacin can reduce fatty deposits in the skin and prevent cholesterol accumulations in the arteries, thus preventing the development of atherosclerosis. It greatly improves circulation.

Mega-doses of niacin, such as those recommended by Dr. Hoffer, should be taken only with a doctor's supervision. Normal preventive daily doses should not exceed 100-200 mg. During stress, this dose can be doubled. Remember, however, that each time one singular B-vitamin dosage is increased, the dosages of the other vitamins from the B-complex should be raised, too.

• *Pangamic acid (vitamin B₁₅)* is extremely valuable in preventing premature aging because it not only stimulates and improves oxygen metabolism and supply to the cells, but also reduces random oxidation in the cells. It is involved in protein metabolism, helps to protect against exogenous toxins through improved oxygenation, lowers serum cholesterol, and prevents fatty degeneration of the liver. It is specifically valuable in protecting against poisoning by carbon monoxide, because it increases the body's tolerance to hypoxia, or lowered oxygen supply. Carbon monoxide (the most damaging part of polluted air) interferes with the body's ability to effectively utilize oxygen, and, thus, can contribute to a host of serious health problems and premature aging. B_{15} can effectively help to protect the body from the damaging effects of carbon monoxide. Daily adult dosage is 50 to 150 mg.

• *PABA and Folic Acid.* These two B vitamins play a key role in preventing premature aging. They are both involved in keeping sex glands working effectively, increasing virility and vitality. Folic acid is essential for protein synthesis, production of DNA and RNA, and cell division and regeneration. PABA has some anti-oxidant activity. It also protects against exposure to ozone. Both PABA and folic acid are also anti-stress factors and anti-graying agents—together with pantothenic acid, and other B vitamins, they can prevent graying of the hair, and, sometimes, even reverse it.

• *Pyrodoxine (vitamin B_6)* can help to keep the libido at a high level despite advancing age. It is essential for the synthesis and proper action of DNA and RNA. It aids in protein and fat metabolism and activates many enzyme systems. It helps in healthy functions of the brain, nervous system, and reproductive organs. It can relieve premenstrual edema and cramps.

There are many other B vitamins which I didn't mention in the above list, but these are the vitamins from the B-complex that are directly involved in keeping you younger longer.

The best natural sources of B vitamins are brewer's yeast; whole grains; fresh, raw wheat germ; raw nuts; sunflower seeds; green leafy vegetables; rice polishings; peas and beans; milk and milk products. Incorporating these foods in your optimum diet will help to assure that you obtain all these vital nutrients and keep you younger longer. If B vitamins are taken in supplementary form, make sure that you take a multiple B-complex tablet that contains all the B vitamins, preferably one that is 100% natural, made from concentrated yeast or rice polishings.

Synthetic B-complex tablets should not be taken by relatively young and healthy persons in potencies over 25 mg. (or 25 mcg.) of each vitamin. Older persons, those over 50, can take one 50-strength B-complex tablet a day.

BREWER'S YEAST

The single most potent rejuvenative food is brewer's yeast. Here are some of its miraculous health-building, disease-preventing, and life-prolonging properties:

- It is the richest natural source of all B vitamins. As I reported previously, most of the B vitamins —particularly B_1, B_2, B_3, B_6, PABA, folic acid, and pantothenic acid—are specific rejuvenators and life prolongators.
- It is one of the best sources of zinc, which is of specific importance for the healthy function of male sex organs and for the prevention of prostate disorders.
- It contains a huge amount of the highest quality proteins (up to 40-50% of its weight!)—3 times more than meat. Yeast proteins are superior in quality to those in meat or many other animal sources.
- It is the richest natural source of the nucleic acids, RNA and DNA. Nucleic acids are considered to be *the* rejuvenative factor, contributing to the

healthy function of all the cells in the body, and keeping the mental and physical processes at the peak of their youthful efficiency. Although I do not advise taking nucleic acids in isolated form, nucleic acid in brewer's yeast is safe, easily assimilated, and harmless.

* Brewer's yeast is the best natural source of selenium, a very important aging-preventive mineral. (Read about the life-prolonging properties of selenium later in this chapter.)

Brewer's yeast is available in powder form, flakes, or tablets. If consumed regularly, it can help to keep you young by preventing the degenerative diseases and halting the aging processes. Of all the various edible yeasts available on the market, true brewer's yeast is the best for keeping you younger longer; not primary yeast, not yeast number so or so, but plain brewer's yeast.

LECITHIN

Lecithin is an organic phosphorized fat substance, the chief constituent of brain and nerve tissues. Close to 20 percent of brain substance is made up of lecithin. Lecithin is also present in abundance in the endocrine glands, especially the gonads — both male and female. Pituitary and pineal glands contain lecithin. The pineal gland is richer in lecithin than any other part of the body. Lecithin is also an essential component of semen, and a sufficient supply is necessary for normal semen production. Lecithin has been used successfully by some doctors to treat male sexual debility and glandular exhaustion. They claim that lecithin improves virility and prevents impotency.

Lecithin can also be a great life saver by helping to prevent heart disease caused by atherosclerosis. Lecithin destroys cholesterol deposits in the arteries, thus lessening the chance of a heart attack.

Dr. Lester M. Morrison, senior attending physician at Los Angeles County General Hospital, says that lecithin is "one of our most powerful weapons against disease." In the treatment of heart disease, Dr. Morrison "found lecithin to give the most rewarding results ..." He even found that lecithin not only can prevent atherosclerosis, but in many instances, *reverse* it, making old hardened arteries younger. This is significant, since many scientists believe that "you are as young as your arteries." If lecithin can help to keep your arteries from aging, it can help you to stay younger longer.

Lecithin is truly a miraculous food supplement. It is a rich source of many rejuvenative food elements, such as vitamins E, D, and K, essential fatty acids, and especially choline and inositol, two B vitamins that are involved in helping to prevent the aging processes. Choline and inositol are perfect fat-dissolving agents.

As you can see, lecithin is a very important anti-aging superfood. It can help dissolve both cholesterol accumulations and fat deposits, and thus prevent heart disease, our life-shortener number one.

Note: Recommended daily adult dosage is 1 tsp. of granules. If large doses of lecithin are taken, calcium should be added to the diet (bone-meal, dolomite, or calcium lactate tablets) to balance the excess phosphorus obtained from the lecithin.

MINERALS

Just as there are specific vitamins with scientifically proven age-retarding and life-prolonging properties, there are several minerals that are specific in helping to control the aging processes and keeping you younger longer.

SELENIUM is the number one life-extension mineral. Actually, it is a trace element, since it appears in natural foods only in minute trace amounts.

Selenium is a powerful antioxidant and free-radical deactivator. When taken together with the other major natural antioxidants and free-radical deactivators, vitamins E and C, selenium enhances their efficiency. It is a co-factor in the enzyme gluthionine peroxidase which converts harmful lipid peroxides (before they change into free-radicals) to harmless hydroxy acids which can be easily eliminated from the system. Selenium is also a detoxicant. It neutralizes the toxic effect of mercury and helps protect the body from damage by mercury poisoning. Selenium can help in regeneration of the liver after damage, especially by cirrhosis.

Because of its ability to prevent the development of free-radicals and even deactivate the existing free-radicals, selenium is considered to be an effective protector against certain forms of cancer, specifically breast cancer, which is causatively linked to free-radicals.

Famous researcher, Raymond Schamberger, was able to lower the incidence of cancer in mice by 50 percent by adding selenium to their food. Gerhard N. Schrauzer, at the University of California in San Diego, was able to demonstrate an even greater drop in mammary cancer incidence with selenium supplements — from 82 percent to 10 percent.

Several studies correlate low cancer rates to high selenium content in the soil and food grown in such soil. Unfortunately, much of the soil in the United States is low in selenium; consequently, the American diet is relatively deficient in selenium as compared with some other countries. For example, in the Philippines, the average daily intake of selenium is 189 mcg. as compared to the average American intake of only 68 mcg. The incidence of female breast cancer in America is four times higher than in the Philippines. The average dietary intake of selenium among the Japanese is 287 mcg., and the breast cancer rate is five times lower than in the United States. A high selenium intake also reduces the incidence of leukemia and cancers of the stomach, colon, prostate, liver, and lung, as Dr. Raymond Schamberger's studies show.

Selenium, however, is toxic in large doses. Those who wish to take selenium in supplementary form should take no more than 100-150 mcg. a day. My usual recommended preventive dose is only 50 mcg. a day. Of course, selenium from food sources is completely harmless. The best natural sources of selenium are: brewer's yeast (not primary-grown yeast), sea foods, kelp, garlic, onions, and grains and vegetables grown in selenium-rich soils. The most concentrated food source is a special high-selenium yeast, which is available from health food stores.

ZINC is another mineral which is directly involved in keeping you younger longer. Zinc is essential for the formation of RNA and DNA, and for the synthesis of protein. It is involved in many enzymatic processes and hormone activities, especially in the reproductive hormones. Zinc is essential for normal growth and development of the sex organs, and for healthy function of the prostate gland. It promotes healing of virtually every disease and is especially helpful in the healing of burns and wounds. It also stimulates the immune system, breaks down fatty deposits, and lowers cholesterol. As you can see, zinc can contribute to a lengthened life by preventing and helping to correct age-related diseases that shorten life.

One unique way zinc is directly involved in retarding premature aging is its ability to neutralize the damaging effects of excess copper on various body functions. Although copper is an essential mineral, we usually get more than enough of it, sometimes excessively so, primarily because of copper piping used in plumbing. Excessive copper actually acts as a catalyst to cause rapid peroxidation of lipids, and, thus, increases the proliferation of free-radicals. It can also lead to hardening of the arteries, kidney damage, schizophrenia, early senility, and other disorders of aging. Zinc, on the other hand, neutralizes most of the adverse effects of copper. If the diet contains sufficient zinc — the normal zinc-to-copper ratio should be 14 to 1 — the copper is neutralized and cannot accomplish its usual harmful effects.

The best natural sources of zinc are wheat bran and fresh wheat germ, pumpkin seeds, sunflower seeds, brewer's yeast, nuts, milk, eggs, onions, garlic, green vegetables, and some sea foods. Zinc in grains is not easily available for assimilation because it is chemically bound to phytins. This bond is broken down by the fermentation process, as for example in sourdough bread, and also by sprouting.

If zinc is taken in supplementary form, which is easily available from any health food store, the dosage should be between 15 and 25 mg. a day. Those who have digestive problems and cannot assimilate supplementary minerals should take zinc, as well as other minerals, in a chelated form. Chelated minerals are available in most health food stores.

CALCIUM and MAGNESIUM are two other minerals which are vital for almost every body function, and an adequate amount of both is an absolute must for optimum health and long life. Calcium and magnesium work synergistically to reduce stress. They also help to keep cholesterol levels down.

The American diet, with its excess phosphorus (from meat and refined grains) is usually lacking in calcium and magnesium, which is a contributing factor to our epidemic of such disorders as osteoporosis, osteoarthritis, diabetes, tooth decay, and heart disease.

It would be wise to supplement your diet with extra calcium and magnesium. 1,000 mg. of calcium and 500 mg. of magnesium would be an adequate supplementary dose. Dolomite is a good natural source of both calcium and magnesium. Unfortunately, there have been some reports that certain brands of dolomite contain excessive amounts of lead. Before you take dolomite, request from the manufacturers of your particular brand the analysis concerning pollutants in their product. Other supplementary sources of calcium would be calcium lactate or calcium gluconate, which can be balanced with appropriate amounts of magnesium oxide (500 mg. of magnesium for each 1,000 mg. of calcium).

MOLYBDENUM is another micro-nutrient that has been largely overlooked as an important factor in preventing the aging processes. Molybdenum is essential in several body functions that are directly related to aging. Like zinc, molybdenum is an antagonist to copper; thus, it can protect from copper poisoning. It is also an integral part of certain enzymes, particularly those involved in controlling the oxidation processes. Molybdenum is a part of the xanthine oxidase enzyme which helps in preventing lipid peroxidation. It can also help protect the organs and tissues of the body, especially the stomach and esophagus, from cancer. It can improve sexual functioning in older men. Molybdenum is also needed for proper carbohydrate metabolism, which usually slows down with age.

The best natural sources of molybdenum are whole grain cereals, especially brown rice, millet, and buckwheat; brewer's yeast; legumes; and naturally hard water. Molybdenum supplements are now available in health food stores. Doses of 50 to 100 mcg. daily are considered to be safe.

Again, I wish to emphasize, just as I did following the section on vitamins, that although I listed here only a few specific minerals and trace elements which possess unique anti-aging and life-prolonging properties, *all* minerals and micro-nutrients essential to human nutrition should be included in any supplementary program designed to optimize nutrition, improve health, prevent premature aging, and prolong life. All supplements, both vitamins and minerals, work synergistically, and are, therefore, most effective when taken together.

14

THE TRUE FOUNTAINS OF YOUTH:
Optimum Nutrition, Exercise, Relaxation and Positive Attitude

In preceding chapters, I have presented to you the health and longevity secrets from around the world — that "work." I have deliberately left out all controversial rejuvenation methods, such as cellular injections, gland and organ transplants, toxic "youth drugs," hormones, synthetic antioxidants, and other alleged life-extension drugs and surgical approaches. Only those methods are reported that are scientifically or empirically proven.

If we summarize what has been said throughout the book so far, we will find that basically

- You are as young as your glands
- You are as young as your cells
- You are as young as your collagen and other connective tissues
- You are as young as your digestive and assimilative system
- You are as young as your arteries
- You are as young as your mind

But in order to keep your glands and organs young and efficient, your digestive tract free from decay and putrefaction, your cells well oxygenated, healthy and vital, your collagen elastic, your arteries open and free from cholesterol, and your mind clear and efficient, *you have to feed your body with the highest quality nutrition* — nutrition which will supply your glands, organs, and tissues with adequate amounts of all the *nutrients* essential for normal, healthy, and efficient functioning. Which leads us to the conclusion that

THE ULTIMATE SECRET OF STAYING YOUNG IS STAYING HEALTHY

And, the secret of staying healthy is closely tied to proper nutrition. My search for the secrets of long life leads me to the inevitable conclusion that one of the *True Fountains of Youth is Optimum Nutrition.* More and more researchers of the new science of Gerontology agree with me.

It is generally agreed, of course, that the state of your mind has a determining influence on your health. But even the state of your mind — your attitudes, your mental capacities and your ability to cope with severe emotional conflicts and stresses, the ability to deal with traumatic experiences or losses — depends to a great extent on the quality of your nutrition. "A sound mind can only dwell in a sound body," said the old Romans. The modern sciences of psychosomatics and nutrition have proven that the Romans were right. As Dr. Henry C. Sherman, of Columbia University, said, "not only can human life be extended, but also youthfulness can be preserved, and the extended life made more useful, by the right selection of foods." Most nutritionists are in complete agreement that chronic malnutrition is one of the prime causes of premature aging, and that optimum nutrition is imperative for optimum health and long life.

What Constitutes OPTIMUM NUTRITION?

Now that we have agreed that optimum nutrition is absolutely necessary for the maintenance of optimum health and the prevention of disease and premature aging, the question is: *what is optimum nutrition, or what constitutes the optimum diet for optimum health?*

There are those who believe that the so-called "four basic food groups" will assure optimum nutrition. There are those who advocate a high-animal-protein diet, with lots of meat. There are vegetarians, lacto-vegetarians, lacto-ovo-vegetarians, vegans, fruitarians, and even breatherians. There are those who condemn all seeds and grains; those who eat seeds, but not grains; those who eat only vegetables that grow above the ground; those who condemn honey; and those who consider tomatoes and onions to be poisonous. There are those who advocate taking vitamins and food supplements — and there are those who claim that all added vitamins are harmful, and you should get all your vitamins from the food you eat. There are those who advocate eating only raw foods; then there are those who consider the discovery of fire the greatest boon to man's nutrition.

Now, perhaps, you may think that I am trying to be funny — that I am exaggerating the great variety of beliefs and fads about man's proper diet. Believe me, this is just a very small sample of what is actually going on. In my capacity as a nutrition consultant, lecturer, and traveler, I never cease to be amazed at the unbelievable confusion in this field. I have found that not only the average person, but also the well-read, well-educated veteran health seekers are thoroughly confused on the most vital questions related to nutrition and to the right ways and means of attaining optimum health. The more they read, the more lectures they attend — the more confused they become. Every book, every lecturer, and every "authority" gives them different answers and points out different roads to glorious health and long life. Truly, it's a jungle out there!

I have spent half a century—a lifetime—of research to find out the *real* truth regarding optimum nutrition for optimum health. As a member of the International Society for Research on Diseases of Civilization and Environment, the most respected nutrition research organization in the world, which was founded by Dr. Albert Schweitzer, I have continuous access to the most up-to-date and most reliable findings regarding nutrition and its effect on man's health, which are reported by hundreds of research scientists from 75 countries. I have also traveled in many countries around the world, and have studied the eating and living habits of many natives, particularly those known for their exceptional health and longevity, as is reported in this book. On the basis of this extensive research and personal and clinical experience, I have made my conclusions which I am sharing with you in this book. *The Airola Diet for Optimum Health and Long Life*, presented below, is not based on my own personal, subjective beliefs, likes or wishful thinking, but on reliable scientific sources and corroborated by overwhelming empirical and scientific evidence. This diet has not only the greatest potential for building health, preventing disease, and maintaining health, but also for preventing premature aging and keeping you younger longer.*

---

*) For a complete, detailed description of the AIROLA DIET FOR OPTIMUM HEALTH, see my books: *How to Get Well*, and *The Airola Diet and Cookbook*. Available at all health food stores, or from the publisher: Health Plus Publishers, P.O. Box 22001, Phoenix, AZ 85028. See back cover of this book for details.

TEN BASIC PRINCIPLES OF
OPTIMUM NUTRITION

The Airola Diet for Optimum Health, Maximum Vitality, and Long Life

1. *Your Optimum Diet should be made up of these three basic food groups (in this order of importance):*
   (1) Seeds, nuts, grains, and legumes
   (2) Vegetables
   (3) Fruits

Seeds, grains, and nuts are the most important and the most potent foods of all. Their nutritional value is unsurpassed by any other food. Eaten mostly raw, but also cooked, they contain all the important nutrients essential for human growth, sustenance of health, and prevention of disease and premature aging.

All seeds and grains are beneficial, but sesame seeds, sunflower seeds, millet, buckwheat, rice, rye, and oats are especially recommended. All beans and peas are useful, as are all nuts. Almonds are excellent sources of complete protein, as well as unsaturated fats, minerals, and other vital nutrients.

Sprouting increases the nutritional value of seeds and grains and makes even those grains that do not contain the ideal levels of all the essential amino acids, into a better protein food. Wheat, mung beans, alfalfa seeds, and soybeans make excellent sprouts. However, my research indicates that wheat, mung bean, and soybean sprouts should be lightly cooked or steamed before eating.

Grains are best eaten in cooked form. Cooked millet, buckwheat, oats, and rice make tasty, nutritious cereals. Rye makes an excellent sourdough bread (see Chapter 3 for the value of soured lactic-acid foods).

Vegetables are the next most important food in the Airola Optimum Diet. Most vegetables contain complete proteins of high quality. They are also an excellent source of minerals, vitamins, and enzymes. Most vegetables can be eaten raw in the form of salads. Some vegetables, such as potatoes, yams, squashes, spinach, cabbage and green beans, should be cooked. Generous use of garlic, onions, culinary herbs, and natural spices is recommended.

Fruits, like vegetables, are excellent sources of vitamins, minerals, and enzymes. Fruits are a cleansing food. All fruits must be eaten fresh, *in season.* Out of season, some dried fruits such as raisins, prunes, figs, or apricots can be used.

Roughly, one food group should supply the bulk of each of the three meals: fruits for breakfast; seeds, nuts, or cereals for lunch; and vegetables for dinner. (See Health Menu at the end of this section.)

2. *Eat mostly raw, living foods.*

At least 65-70% of your diet should consist of foods in their natural, uncooked state. Numerous studies have demonstrated the superiority of raw, living foods both for the maintenance of health and for the prevention of disease. It has been shown, for example, that you need only one-half of the amount of protein in your diet *if you eat protein foods raw instead of cooked.*

Don't be a raw-food fanatic, however. A certain amount of cooked foods (30-35% of the total diet) will not hurt you, as it, certainly, does not seem to hurt the Hunza people, who are considered to be the healthiest people in the world, with the average life expectancy of 85-90 years, and whose daily staples include such cooked foods as chapati, cereals, and soups.

If you live in an ideal tropical or subtropical climate —man's natural habitat—where fresh vegetables and fruits are available year round, you can live on raw foods almost exclusively. In colder northern regions, a certain amount of cooked food in the form of cereals, bread, potatoes, beans, peas, etc. should be added to the diet.

Speaking of raw versus cooked foods, certain foods are actually better cooked. Grains should always be cooked because raw grains cannot be effectively digested by the human digestive system. Minerals and trace elements in raw grains are chemically bound to phytins; this bond is broken by cooking. Also some vegetables such as spinach, rhubarb, asparagus, and vegetables of the cabbage family, are better eaten cooked. Cooking leaches out or destroys oxalic acid and other toxic factors in these vegetables.

3. Eat only natural foods.

Your foods should be whole, unprocessed, and unrefined, and be organically grown in fertile soil. They should preferably be grown in your own environment and eaten in *their season*.

That your health and longevity are in direct relationship to the *naturalness* of the foods you eat is a well established scientific fact. You have seen in the earlier chapters of this book that where natives eat a diet of natural, whole, unprocessed and unrefined foods, they enjoy superior health, absence of disease, and a long life. When "civilization" enters their lives in the form of denatured, refined, processed, man-made foods, disease becomes rampant among them and their life expectancy drops.

Natural foods are foods that are grown in fertile soils without chemical fertilizers and sprays, and are consumed in their *natural state*, with all the nutrients that nature put in them intact — *nothing removed and nothing added.*

4. Eat only poison-free foods.

Almost all commercially sold food today contains chemicals, which are either used in food producing or added during processing or packing. Some of these poisons cannot be washed off because they are *systemic*, that is, they penetrate the whole fruit or vegetable. The only solution seems to be to grow your own food or buy certified organically grown food. Many health food stores and natural food co-ops sell such produce.

5. Special complementary foods.

Your three basic health-building foods can be complemented with the following foods, if desired:

A. **Milk.** The value of milk in human nutrition has been highly disputed. Some authorities claim that milk is an excellent—indeed, perfect—food for man. Others insist that "milk is for calves," that it is a poison for man, causing mucus, allergies, etc.

The answer to the milk controversy is simple: milk is an excellent health food for those whose ancestors herded dairy animals and traditionally lived on a lactose-rich diet (milk, cheese, butter). These people are genetically programmed to digest milk well, and their intestines contain plenty of the milk-digesting enzyme, *lactase*. Most white Americans of European ancestry fall into this group.

Those whose ancestors never or seldom used milk as a major element in their diet are usually intolerant to milk because their intestines do not contain sufficient lactase. Most American Blacks, Chinese, Japanese, Eskimos, or American Indians fall into this group. They should avoid milk completely.

The best way to use milk is in its soured form: as yogurt, kefir, acidophilus milk, or regular clabbered milk or buttermilk. Soured milks are superior to sweet milk because they are in a predigested form and very easily assimilated. They also help to maintain a healthy intestinal flora and prevent intestinal putrefaction and constipation. As you have seen in Chapters 1 and 4, most people known for their excellent health—Bulgarians, Swedes, Finns, Russians, and Caucasians—consume large amounts of soured milk.

Goat's or sheep's milk is superior to cow's milk as a food for humans. Homemade cottage cheese, some natural cheese, and a small amount of butter can be added to the diet.

B. **Cold-pressed vegetable oils.** High quality, fresh, cold-pressed, crude and unrefined vegetable oils can be used in a very moderate quantity. The average daily amount should not exceed 2 teaspoons.

Make sure oils are genuinely *cold-pressed*, and fresh, *not rancid*. Most oils, even those sold in health food stores, are *not* cold-pressed, even when the label says they are. The only oils likely to be actually cold-pressed, are olive oil and sesame seed oil. Oils must never be used in cooking or frying. Use them only in un-heated, raw state as in salad dressings, dips, etc.

C. **Honey.** Natural, raw, unheated, unfiltered, and unprocessed honey is the only sweetener allowed in the Airola Optimum Diet. Honey possesses miraculous nutritional and medicinal properties. As I have mentioned in previous chapters, most centenarians in Russia, Bulgaria, and Abkhazia use honey liberally in their diets.

Honey is especially beneficial in the diets of older people and children. It increases calcium retention in the system, helps to prevent nutritional anemia, and is beneficial in heart, kidney, and liver disorders, colds, poor circulation, and complexion problems.

6. *Fortify your diet with vitamins, minerals, and food supplements.*

Although, ideally, you should obtain all your vitamins from the foods you eat, today this is almost impossible. Due to vitamin-, protein-, and enzyme-destroying practices of food producing and food processing industries, our modern-day foods, not only those you buy at your supermarket, but even those from your health food store, are nutritionally inferior to the foods your grandparents ate two or three generations ago. Today's grains and vegetables are grown on depleted soils with the help of artificial fertilizers, and they are nutritionally inferior to organically grown foods. But even organically grown foods today are raised in a polluted atmosphere, are watered with polluted waters, and contain residues of toxic atmospheric fallout. The prime purpose of food supplements is to fill in the nutritional gaps produced by faulty eating habits and nutritionally inferior foods.

There is another reason for supplementing your Optimum Diet with extra vitamins and other nutrients. Many of these substances have protective properties against some of today's most toxic environmental factors. They can help protect you from the harmful effects of poisonous additives and residues in your food, water, and air.

As an effective insurance against nutritional deficiencies and protection against the harmful effects of our increasingly toxic environment, I recommend that adults take daily the following specific protective foods and natural vitamin and mineral supplements (some of these have already been mentioned in Chapter 13):

Brewer's yeast — 2-3 tablespoons of powder, flakes, or equivalent in tablets

Kelp — 2-3 tablets, or ½ teaspoon of granules

Lecithin — 1 teaspoon of granules

Vitamin C — 3,000-5,000 mg.

Vitamins A & D — (10,000 A and 400 D per capsule) 2-3 capsules. This must be a 100% natural product made from fish oils.

Vitamin E, mixed tocopherols — 600 I.U. to 1,200 I.U.

Vitamin B-complex with B_{12}, the highest available potency of 100% natural B-complex from yeast concentrate—4-6 tablets (Note: the usual strength of 100% natural B-complex does not exceed 10 mg. for most major B's.)

Calcium and magnesium tablets — 2-3 tablets

Zinc — 15 mg. for women and young men, and 25-30 mg. for men over fifty

Selenium — 50-100 mcg.

B_{15} — 50-100 mg.

All supplements should be taken with meals.

Please understand that the above suggested list of supplements is only a very general outline of the supplementary needs of the average individual. However, there are no average or common individuals, biochemically speaking. The individual needs for nutrients vary considerably from person to person. Therefore, it would be wise, especially if you suffer from one or more conditions of ill health (and who doesn't) that you enlist the help of a good nutrition consultant or nutritionally-oriented doctor who can help to work out an individualized supplementary program for your specific needs.

If you wish to know more about vitamins and supplements, their functions, deficiency symptoms, differences between natural and synthetic, and specific dosages for specific conditions of ill health, please refer to my books, *How To Get Well*, and *The Airola Diet and Cookbook*. The recommended maintenance doses of supplements for different age groups are listed in Chapter 9 of *Everywoman's Book*.

7. *Avoid an excess of protein in your diet.*

The Optimum Diet of three basic foods—seeds, nuts and grains; vegetables; and fruits — supplemented with the special super-foods and food supplements named above, will assure you an adequate supply of all required nutrients for optimum health and long life, *including sufficient amounts of complete high quality proteins.* A small amount of eggs, fish, or meat may be added to this basic diet, if desired — particularly fish in coastal areas, or meat in far northern regions with long winters—*but their inclusion is not necessary.* In temperate, sub-tropical or tropical climates, the highest level of health and longevity can be best achieved and maintained without meat.

A high-animal-protein diet is definitely detrimental to health and may cause or contribute to the development of many of our most common diseases, such as arthritis, heart disease, cancer, osteoporosis, schizophrenia, kidney damage, and severe vitamin and mineral deficiencies, as proven in extensive clinical studies. A high-protein diet also causes premature aging and lowers life expectancy. (Well-documented evidence regarding the dangers of a high-protein diet can be found in my books, *Everywoman's Book,* and *The Airola Diet and Cookbook;* also in Chapter 8 of this book.)

8. *Drink pure, natural water.*

The best water for drinking is pure, natural, uncontaminated spring, river, or well water. Avoid prolonged drinking of distilled water. Dozens of actual studies from the United States, England, Europe, and Japan, show that the minerals in naturally-hard water are important to man's nutrition. Studies show that where people drink naturally-hard (highly mineralized) water, they have less heart disease, less tooth decay, less diabetes, and less arteriosclerosis. Minerals, as they are naturally present in drinking water, have been an essential part of man's mineral nutrition since the beginning of his life on this planet.

Contrary to what some "experts" claim, inorganic minerals in natural water *are* effectively absorbed and utilized in human metabolism. We need both organic and inorganic minerals. Foods supply organic minerals, and water inorganic minerals. (See Chapters 3 and 8.)

9. Cultivate the following health-promoting eating habits:

- Eat only when really hungry.
- Eat slowly and in a relaxed atmosphere.
- Eat several small meals during the day in preference to a few large meals.
- Do not mix too many foods at the same meal—the less mixing, the better the digestion.
- Do not mix raw fruits and raw vegetables at the same meal—they are incompatible in regard to digestive enzymes, and mixing them will only result in poor digestion.
- When protein-rich foods are eaten with other foods, eat the protein-rich foods *first*. It is wrong to eat a large vegetable salad in the beginning of the meal, and then continue with protein food. For effective digestion, protein requires lots of hydrochloric acid, which is more plentiful in the beginning of the meal when the stomach is empty. This pattern of eating is followed by all people known for their exceptional health and long life.
- Finally, practice *systematic undereating*. Systematic undereating is the number one health and longevity secret. Studies of centenarians around the world show that they are moderate eaters throughout their lives. You never see an obese centenarian. Overeating, on the other hand, is one of the main causes of disease and premature aging. Overeating, and particularly overindul-

gence in proteins, is especially dangerous to older people who are less active and have a slowed metabolism. *The unbelievable fact is that the less you eat, the less hungry you feel, because the food is more efficiently digested and better utilized.* At an important symposium on the relationship between nutrition and longevity, a highly competent group of international experts in the field agreed that the restriction of food intake to a point that would be considered undernutrition by contemporary standards lengthens the life and improves the health by reducing the susceptibility to the diseases of aging (*Journal of Clinical Nutrition*, August, 1972).

As Benjamin Franklin said, "To lengthen the life, lessen the meals." My own dictum on the subject goes as follows: "A man's belt length determines his life's length: the longer the belt—the shorter the life."

10. Avoid the following health destroyers and life shorteners:

This is the list of *do nots*, the things you must avoid if you wish to achieve optimum health. These are scientifically proven to be powerfully destructive health and longevity factors:

- All tobacco. Smoking causes cancer and heart disease and, thus, shortens life. It also causes premature aging, wrinkles, and dull, lifeless complexion.
- Coffee, tea, chocolate, cola drinks, and other soft drinks.
- Excessive use of salt.
- Excessive consumption of alcohol.
- Harmful spices: black and white pepper, mustard, white vinegar.

- White sugar and white flour, and everything made with them.
- All processed, refined, canned, or factory-made foods.
- All rancid foods, such as rancid seeds, nuts, oils, and rancid wheat germ. (Wheat germ is rancid if it is older than one week to ten days after it is milled.)
- All chemical drugs (except in emergencies, prescribed by a doctor).
- All toxic household and environmental chemicals: garden sprays; air fresheners; household chemicals and cleaners; detergents (use soap flakes); hair sprays; chemically cleaned or treated clothes, beds, or wallpaper; bug and fly killers; etc.

YOUR STAY-YOUNGER-LONGER MENU

Based on the information presented in this chapter, your daily menu for a health-building and rejuvenating diet should look something like this:

Upon Arising: Glass of pure water—plain, or with choice of freshly squeezed citrus juice: ½ lime, ¼ lemon, ½ grapefruit, or 1 orange to a glass of water.

Or: Large cup of warm herb tea sweetened with honey. Choice of rose hips, peppermint, camomile, or any of your favorite herbs. Or you may choose one of the following rejuvenative and life-extending herbs: ginseng, gotu kola, licorice, damiana or sarsaparilla.

Or: Glass of freshly made fruit juice from any available fruit or berry in season: apple, pineapple, orange, cherry, pear, etc. The juice should be diluted with water, half and half. No canned or frozen juices—the juice must be freshly made just before drinking.

After this morning drink, you should walk for one hour in fresh air, combining your walk with deep-breathing exercises and all the calisthenics you can manage to squeeze in. If you have a garden, or if you live on a farm, you should get in a couple of hours of hard physical labor.

Upon returning from your long walk or garden work, and after a cold shower to wash the perspiration away, you are now, *but not before*, ready for breakfast.

Breakfast: Fresh fruits, preferably organically grown: apple, orange, banana, grapes, grapefruit, or any available berries and fruits, *in season.*

Cup of yogurt, kefir, or homemade soured milk, preferably goat's milk (see Chapter 3 for recipes and instructions).

Handful of raw nuts, such as almonds, or sesame seeds. Nuts and seeds can be freshly crushed or ground in your seed grinder (sold in health food stores) and sprinkled over yogurt.

Or: Bowl of oatmeal, with 4-6 soaked prunes, or 2-3 figs, and a handful of unsulfured raisins. (This choice only if cereals are not eaten for lunch.)

Glass of raw unpasteurized milk, preferably goat's milk, or yogurt.

Midmorning
Snack: One apple, banana, or other fruit.

Lunch: Bowl of whole-grain cereal, such as millet cereal, buckwheat cereal, whole rice, or oatmeal. Any other available whole-grain cereals, such as triticale, barley, brown rice, or corn, can be used.

Large glass of raw milk, preferably goat's milk.

The cereal can be eaten with home-made applesauce.

Or: Bowl of freshly prepared vegetable soup or any other cooked vegetable dish, such as potatoes, yams, squash, beans and corn tortillas. Kelp, sea salt, cold-pressed vegetable oil, and fresh butter, as well as any of the natural herbs can be used for seasoning.

1-2 slices of whole-grain bread, preferably sourdough rye bread (see Chapter 2).

1 or 2 slices of natural cheese. Never use processed cheeses.

Mid-afternoon: Glass of fresh fruit or vegetable juice.

Or: Cup of your favorite herb tea, sweetened with honey.

Or: One apple, banana, pear, or other available fruit.

Dinner: Large bowl of fresh, green vegetable salad. Use any and all available vegetables—preferably those in season—including tomatoes, avocados, and alfalfa seed sprouts. Carrots, shredded red beets, and onions should be staples in every salad. Raw garlic, if your social life permits. Salad should be attractively prepared and served with homemade dressing of lemon juice (or apple cider vinegar) and cold-pressed vegetable oil, seasoned with herbs, garlic powder, a little sea salt, cayenne pepper, etc. But vegetables can also be placed attractively on the plate without mixing them into a salad, and eaten one at a time—this is, by far, the superior way of eating vegetables.

2 or 3 middle sized boiled or baked potatoes in jackets. Prepared cooked vegetable course, if desired: eggplant, artichoke, sweet potatoes, yams, squash, or other vegetables. Use kelp powder or sea salt sparingly for seasoning; also any or all of the usual garden herbs.

Fresh homemade cottage cheese, or 1-2 slices of natural cheese.

1 pat fresh butter or 1 tsp. of cold-pressed vegetable oil (can be used on salad, soup, or potatoes).

Glass of yogurt or other soured milk.

Or: Any of the recommended lunch choices, if fresh vegetable salad is eaten at lunch.

Bedtime
Snack: Glass of fresh milk, or nut-milk, or seed-milk (made in electric liquifier from raw seeds or raw nuts and water

— milk can be added or not, according to preference) with a tablespoon of honey.

Or: Glass of yogurt with brewer's yeast.

Or: Cup of your favorite herb tea with a slice of whole grain bread with butter and a slice of natural cheese.

Or: One apple.

Vital points to remember

1. The above menu is only a very general outline, a skeleton, around which an individual diet of optimum nutrition should be built. It can be followed as it is, of course — I know of thousands of people who live on such a diet and enjoy extraordinary health. But it also can be modified and changed to adapt to your specific requirements and conditions, your country's customs and climate, the availability of foods, your health condition, your preferences, etc.

2. Whatever changes you make, however, keep in mind that the bulk of your diet should consist of seeds, nuts, and grains, and fresh vegetables and fruits, preferably organically grown, and up to 70% of them eaten raw. Eat as great a variety of available foods as possible, but not in the same meal, of course. Do not shun potatoes, avocados, and bananas because you think they are fattening—they are not!

3. The menu for lunch and dinner is interchangeable. One big vegetable meal should be eaten at least once a day. If it is eaten for lunch, some of the lunch suggestions can be eaten for dinner.

4. Remember, when you eat protein-rich foods (cottage cheese, nuts, beans, etc.) together with carbohydrate-rich foods (salads, fruits, etc.)—eat the protein-rich foods *first*, or *together with* carbohydrate-rich foods,

but *not after*. If you follow this advice, your digestion will improve dramatically.

5. Do not drink water with meals. If thirsty, drink between meals, or 15 minutes before meals. Milk and yogurt are foods.

6. If you are taking vitamins and other food supplements, take them *with* meals. Brewer's yeast is best taken on an empty stomach 1 hour before meal, mixed with fruit juice or yogurt.

7. During the transition period from the typical American diet of meat and potatoes most people long for a large variety of tasty dishes, rather than eating simple salads and cereals every day. For them, I've just published my latest book, *The Airola Diet and Cookbook*, which contains over 300 delicious and nutritious recipes.

8. Finally, if you follow this Health Menu *every day of your life* and take all the supplements as recommended in this chapter, you can live a long life and enjoy the highest possible level of health. And be assured that this Optimum Diet will supply you not only with *all* the vitamins, minerals, essential fatty acids, trace elements, enzymes and the other identified and unidentified nutritive substances, but also with an adequate amount of the highest quality proteins you need for optimum health!

Note from the publisher: Those who wish to learn more about the Airola Diet, should read Dr. Airola's most recent book, *The Airola Diet and Cookbook*, published in 1982, which, in addition to the most detailed and comprehensive description of the philosophical and scientific basis for the Airola Diet, also contains over 300 delicious and nutritious recipes, plus Dr. Airola's famous Weight Loss Program, the only reducing diet that can safely take pounds off while improving your health. See back cover for the ordering details.

EXERCISE

The title of this chapter reads: "The True Fountains of Youth: Optimum Nutrition, Exercise, Relaxation and a Positive Attitude." Actually, I should have added "In *reverse* order of importance!" I may shock you by writing this (and coming from the pen of a nutritionist, this is shocking, indeed!) but, as important as nutrition is, I consider the other three of the Fountains of Youth named in the chapter title even more important than nutrition. I hope that when you finish reading this chapter, you will understand why I place them in such an order of priorities.

In one of my magazine articles a couple of years back I said something that has been quoted, misquoted, and misunderstood, and has shocked lots of readers. I said:

"It is better to eat junk foods and exercise a lot, than to eat health foods and not exercise at all!"

The ideal, of course, is to *eat health foods and exercise a lot*. But, I have seen so many well-meaning health faddists who spend all their money on buying expensive health foods and supplements, don't miss a health lecture, and read every new health book that comes off the press—yet, they haven't reached the optimal level of well-being, and some are in a rather poor state of health, *because they never exercise*. On the other hand, we all have acquaintances who horrify us by the way they eat, seemingly violating all the basic rules of healthful eating—yet, they enjoy apparent good health and vitality *because they are what we call physical fitness freaks, exercising at every opportunity.* You see, exercise is so important for optimal well-being, that even if we eat a less nutritious or inadequate diet, the benefits of enhanced metabolism, improved circulation and elimination, and improved lymphatic, nervous, and glandular functions compensate for the dietary inadequacies. But, if we eat the most nutritious diet in the world, organic and all, and take every new vitamin and supplement, but do not get sufficient exercise, health foods and vitamins will do us no good because our bodies will not be able to properly digest and utilize what we eat; nor will we be able to eliminate all the toxins created within the body by sedentary living. The body's vital functions, cell metabolism, nerve and brain activity, digestive and assimilative processes, immune system, glandular and lymphatic activity, blood circulation—all will be negatively affected by a sedentary life without vigorous exercise.

Life is motion. Your body's most important nutritional requirement is not protein, vitamins, enzymes, fats, minerals—it is oxygen! You can live for months without any food, for days without water, but only for a few minutes without oxygen. Nutritionists, in their illustrative description of the body's mechanism, like to compare it to an automobile. "Just as your car runs best on pure, high quality gas, your body requires the highest quality food to run friction-free." This comparison is misleading. The automobile-gas relationship should be compared to the body-*oxygen* relationship. Oxygen is the most important nutrient for every organ and every cell of your body. How can you get enough of it?

I have often referred to the effective and optimal functioning of your body as dependent on special biorhythms or life-cycles, a kind of genetic programming which has been determined and formed as a result of man's adaptation to the historical and traditional circumstances of his environment. One of the environmental circumstances of prehistoric man was his great mobility connected with daily living. To survive and provide nourishment, man had to move a great deal. And this he had to do on his own two legs. Much walking, running, moving about, and lifting was done during most of the day. Consequently, after thousands of years of adaptation to this kind of lifestyle, man's body was genetically programmed and adjusted to function efficiently on the level of oxygen that was generated by such a mobile lifestyle.

Our present lifestyle has eliminated 90 percent of the motion and exercise our bodies used to have. We do not move on our own power any more—cars and airplanes take care of that. We do not need to exercise our muscles to get our food—we simply drive to the supermarket; and even there we use a cart to haul the food back to our car. Such a lifestyle results in a body which isn't getting much oxygen. The level of oxygen absorption is determined by the level of physical exertion. Our sedentary life has led to a chronic oxygen starvation. Our organs, muscles, brain, nerves, which were designed to function at optimum capacity on a certain level of oxygen, now are forced to cope with their tasks on a constant undersupply of this most important nutrient. The consequences are obvious: physical and mental deterioration and a growing amount of disease that has developed since man has adopted his new, sedentary, mechanized lifestyle, with its polluted environment, where he is getting less and less oxygen.

The only way you can bring more oxygen into your system now is by deliberate exercise. With exercise, I do not mean only a few calisthenics in front of your television, or some slow yoga movements—although both can be beneficial in conjunction with more strenuous activity —but vigorous daily exercise such as jogging, running, playing tennis, biking, swimming, etc., which will lead to an accelerated heartbeat and perspiration. Vigorous exercise is needed to bring the maximum amount of oxygen into tissues and organs. Vigorous exercise, and the oxygen it brings into the system, is imperative for the proper functioning of all organs, *especially the all-important lymphatic system.*

Exercise should be done outdoors, in pure, unpolluted air. It breaks my heart to see well-meaning exercise enthusiasts on busy streets or highways running between fume-spewing automobiles, seemingly unaware that they are doing themselves much more harm than good. No better off are all those who are trying to improve their fitness in downtown gyms and spas, where the air is filled with everything conceivable except pure oxygen.

By far, the best form of exercise is brisk walking in fresh, pure air. If you live in a smoggy area, make an effort to get out where the air is pure for your exercise. You don't need fancy spa equipment to exercise. Garden work, games such as tennis, basketball, volleyball, swimming, bicycling, and just plain walking are the best forms of exercise.

Men can engage in exhausting sports such as running and weight lifting, but women should avoid too strenuous forms of exercise. Several recent studies show that excessive participation in strenuous athletics, especially running and weight lifting, can adversely affect a woman's health, cause hormonal imbalances, and consequent menstrual disturbances or amenorrhea (failure to menstruate), pronounced masculineness (disappearance of breasts, hair growth on the face and chest, etc.), and, occasionally, because of hormonal changes (lowered estrogen and elevated male hormone levels caused by strenuous physical activity), a more aggressive, masculine-type personality. I know this information will shock many female readers who are "into" running and heavy athletics. It is unfortunate that the current books on physical fitness and running, which have helped create and popularize the present running fad, fail to warn women regarding the dangers I have just mentioned. They make no distinction between men's and women's exercise needs or preferences. The scientific fact is, however, that male and female glandular systems work quite differently and respond differently to severe physical stresses: while strenuous exercise by a man improves his physique and masculinity by *elevating* the levels of male sex hormones in his body, vigorous and strenuous exercises by a woman actually *lowers* the levels of the female sex hormone, estrogen, which can cause many undesirable, unhealthy, and unpleasant changes in her body.

I admit that the information you've just read here is many years ahead of its time. Although this information has appeared in several leading medical journals, the popular press has been largely silent. However, I predict that within a few years it will become common knowledge as more and more authors and popular magazines will dare to publicize such scientific research.

Lest I am misunderstood, let me clarify: both men and women need adequate exercise in order to enjoy optimum health and well-being. But, because of their inherent anatomical, physiological, and glandular differences, they benefit most from different forms of exercise. The best exercises for women, which do not affect hormonal levels adversely, are walking, dancing, including aerobic dancing, swimming, bicycling, calisthenics, volleyball, all kinds of yoga, especially hatha yoga, and, of course, all kinds of outdoor physical activities which are not too strenuous, such as gardening, etc.

Moderation in all things, including exercise.

There is a vast difference between doing and overdoing. Some overzealous fitness freaks in their desire to shape up, have landed in hospitals with prolapsed organs, sprained ankles, and damaged knees, spines, and even hearts. Weight lifting and long distance running are two especially dangerous fads in the fitness craze. We seem to think that anything worth doing is even better if done in excess. There is also a deeply seated notion in our hardy American psyche that if it hurts, it must be "good for you." In our frenzy for fitness we forget that *moderation* is one all-important criteria which determines when a certain activity is healthful and when it is not.

Finally, use common sense and *simplify!* The current interest in fitness is plagued with a destructive affliction: greedy commercialization. Fitness is now a thirty billion dollar business! It need not be. You don't need fancy, expensive brand shoes, classy spas and workout salons with extravagant exercise equipment. Simple walking, do-it-yourself calisthenics, and garden work are, by far, the best, the safest, and most effective ways to keep physically fit. And, they won't cost you a penny!

RELAXATION

Rest and relaxation are other longevity factors that are of paramount importance. Throughout this book, we emphasize repeatedly that stress is one of the main causes of disease and premature aging. A certain amount of stress is natural, cannot be avoided, and even can be beneficial, *if it is counteracted and balanced by sufficient rest and relaxation.*

The medical consensus today is that mental and

emotional stresses are the prime causes of most degenerative diseases. Mental and emotional stresses, fears, and worries, not only can produce any ailment in the medical book, but will also age you before your time. Anxieties, worries, tensions, hate, envy, jealousy—these are not just undesirable emotional states. They are killers!

Learn to relax! How? In our fast-paced lifestyle, it's not easy. But, it can be done. First, you must be thoroughly convinced that rest and relaxation are absolute *must* factors if you want to stay younger longer. This will motivate you to gradually rearrange your pattern of daily living. Make a habit of having an afternoon nap or siesta. Relax with a good book or enjoyable music now and then. Take a relaxing walk all by yourself. Take mini-vacations as often as possible. Pace yourself. Don't drain yourself of all energy reserves. Conserve and recharge your batteries by occasional pauses and rest periods.

One of the best ways to relax and get the anxieties, tensions, and worries out of your mind is to engage in absorbing hobbies and games: chess, ping pong, painting, music, etc.

Don't make any mistakes about it: rest and relaxation *are* extremely important factors in staying younger longer. Perhaps, the quote taken from the next chapter illustrates best the importance of rest and relaxation. Russia's oldest centenarian, 166-year-old Shirali Mislimov, when asked for his secrets of long life, said:

"I was never in a hurry in my life. He lives long who enjoys life and who bears no jealousy of others, whose heart harbors no malice or anger, who sings a lot and cries a little, who rises and retires with the sun, who likes to work, and who knows how to rest."

For most of us, life is filled with continuous tensions and stresses because we are haunted by the insatiable drive for more "success"—which usually translates into material wealth and power. Even fear of getting old is a stress that can actually contribute to what we fear—getting old prematurely. Don't worry about getting old, just do something to postpone it. And, getting sufficient sleep, rest, and relaxation, is one way you can postpone your aging processes and live younger longer.

POSITIVE ATTITUDE

Now we come to the fourth Fountain of Youth, which is the most important of them all: a positive, health-oriented, youthful state of mind.

As I mentioned a few paragraphs back, a negative attitude towards life and its daily manifestations, anxieties, fears, tension worries, hate, envy, feeling unloved, unneeded, and unfulfilled—such negative emotions are powerfully destructive forces which can break down physical and mental health and bring about every disease in the medical book. Body, mind, and spirit are three inter-related aspects of one human entity; three manifestations of one being. It behooves us to keep our bodies—the temples of the spirit—clean and healthy. An abused and diseased body can affect the mind and spirit negatively. Likewise, an abused mind, filled with emotional stresses and worries, can affect the physical health negatively and break it down. If anything, the power of the mind is even greater than the power of the physical body. A well-balanced, peaceful, harmonious, positive, and health-oriented state of mind is *absolutely imperative* for physical, emotional, and spiritual well-being. One great philosopher, William James, said, "The greatest discovery of our generation is that a human being can alter his life by altering his attitude." And, I will add that it is the greatest discovery of any generation! One of the main causes of failure in any endeavor is the wrong attitude. *With the wrong attitude, you can do everything right and still fail. But with the right attitude, you can do everything wrong and still succeed.* We must build success on attitude, not attitude on success! It is highly significant that God provided man with the power to shape his own thoughts and the privilege of fitting them into any pattern of his choice. A positive mental attitude is the starting point of all riches. And, some of the greatest riches are abundant health and a peaceful, happy, long life.

A positive, health-oriented attitude is the most powerful vaccination for the prevention of virtually any disease. And, not for prevention only: for healing as well! Dwelling on and worrying about disease will only make you worse. Many sick people are hypochondriacs, thinking and talking about disease constantly. In fact, when they gather together, they love to brag about the extent of their misery. If one says that he takes 12 aspirin for his arthritis, the other immediately adds, "That's nothing, I take 22!" If one says, "My uterus has been taken out," the other will not be a loser: "So what?" she says, "I had my uterus, my gallbladder, and my appendix taken out, and half of my breast removed!" This kind of negative disease-oriented attitude, constantly reminding yourself of your imperfections and afflictions, will only reinforce the mental picture of yourself as a sick person, and make healing impossible.

The greatest healing power is within us: it is faith. A positive attitude, faith, belief in your body's own inherent power to heal itself, as well as a reliance on the Greater Power for assistance, are the best medicines known to medical science. *Think* health, *talk* health, *visualize* health, have *faith* in health—*and better health will be your reward!*

Everyone has seen, heard, or read about miraculous healings performed by healers who use such unconventional modalities as the laying on of hands, holy waters, psychic surgery, or prayer. The implication is always that the healer possesses a great healing power. Actually, the great healing power that accomplishes such miraculous healing is within our own bodies; the healer merely helps to release it. Your body is equipped with the most powerful and the most effective healing system known to medical science. Your body is designed to be a self-cleansing, self-repairing, and self-healing mechanism. However, this healing power must be switched on by an act of faith before it can begin to work. Just as your room can be wired with electric power for brilliant light yet will remain in darkness until you switch the power on, so your own great healing capacity will remain untapped and unused, unless it is switched on by the act of faith. When Jesus walked this earth and healed the sick, he used this same power to accomplish his miracles. Everytime he was thanked for miraculous healing, he replied, to the effect: don't thank me—"Thy faith has made thee whole."

Faith is not only the greatest *healing* power, but the greatest power known to man, period. This was realized by Prof. Alexis Carrel, who wrote in his classic book, *Man the Unknown*, that "Prayer is the greatest power known to man." Prayer is an expression of faith. With faith *all* things are possible. Faith not only switches on the healing power within the body, but it releases all the vital energies that can potentiate any goal or accomplishment.

That a positive state of mind and the power of the subconscious can accomplish miraculous healings was demonstrated on a large scale by the famous French healer, Dr. Emile Coué, in the beginning of this century. Dr. Coué achieved a worldwide reputaton by curing thousands of people of every conceivable disease by a most unusual therapy. He sent patients back home, asking them to repeat aloud five times a day the following words: "Every day, in every way, I am getting better, and better, and better!" To skeptics who laughed at such "nonsense," he said, "I don't care what you think, or even whether you believe it or not; just follow my prescription and you will be cured." And, sure enough, those who followed his advice saw to their amazement how every day, in every way, they *did* feel better, and better, and better; how their pains and ailments gradually disappeared; and how they eventually were totally cured. The loud repetition of the words had registered them on the subconscious mind, which "instructed" the healing powers within the body to initiate, and eventually to accomplish, the healing. The phenomenon of faith is actually a conviction on the intuitive, emotional level, as compared to mere belief, which is a conscious, intellectual process.

Relaxation, peace of mind, a positive outlook on life, a contented spirit, an absence of worries and fears, a cheerful disposition, unselfishness, love of mankind and faith in God—these are all powerful health-promoting and life-extending factors which must become a vital part of any successful stay-younger-longer program.

I have mentioned earlier that one of the factors contributing to long life is a youthful state of mind. This is extremely important. We must not allow our child-like enthusiasm, curiosity, adventurous spirit and quest for learning, fun, and excitement get lost as our chronological age advances. In our culture, "old" people are not expected to act young, or child-like. They are locked into old peoples homes, or live in "sun city," are called senior citizens, and are expected to look and act accordingly. So, they begin to dress, act, walk, and think like old people. This kind of attitude definitely contributes to the accelerated aging processes and to premature death.

We should never lose our child-like characteristics as long as we live. There are no scientific reasons whatsoever why we should not preserve youthfulness of spirit and exhibit child-like interest in things around us, keep learning, be curious, imaginative, creative, play games, have fun, dance, sing, and enjoy life to the fullest. This can help us "to die young as late as possible," as one of my favorite anthropologists, Ashley Montagu, who is 75 going on 18, expressed so beautifully.

In short: think and act young—and you will stay younger longer!

In conclusion . . .

Ponce de Leon had traveled around the world searching for the Fountain of Youth. The reason he couldn't find it is because, as this chapter shows, the Fountain of Youth *is within us.* Youth doctors, life-extension researchers, and "longevists" apparently did not learn from Ponce de Leon's mistake. They are searching for the Fountain of Youth in the modern chemical and pharmaceutical laboratories hoping to find the secret of perpetual youth and long life in some mysterious chemical formula. They think they will find a miraculous drug, a little white pill, that will accomplish an amazing miracle of rejuvenation and keep them young and healthy forever. They are destined to the same fate that befell Ponce de Leon who died disappointed and disillusioned, before reaching three-score and ten, because the secret of staying young and living long cannot be found *without*—it is *within* us!

My lifelong study and search for the secrets of optimum health and long life convinced me that the true Fountains of Youth are: optimum nutrition, rest and relaxation, pure air and water, lots of sunshine, avoidance of mental and emotional stresses, plenty of exercise, peace of mind, and a loving, health-oriented, positive attitude with emphasis on spiritual orientation, rather than spending one's energies on the selfish pursuits of material wealth and power. All these factors are within reach of all of us. They can be achieved with proper motivation, change of attitude, will, and dedication. And if you are one of those who is always looking for "scientific references" and "reliable research," I am happy to report that every one of the above-mentioned health-youth-and-longevity factors is substantiated by massive scientific studies and reliable research in reputable research centers around the world.

15

Centenarians Speak ...

Observations, clinical tests, vital statistics, animal studies, laboratory experiments, theories—all these are useful when we are trying to determine the secrets of long life. But nothing is as convincing as the personal testimony of those who have achieved the enviable age of 100 or more years. Let's hear from some of them, in their own words, their secrets of superior health and a long life in youthful vitality.

While in Russia, I met several centenarians. I discovered that they all had a few things in common. They all were moderate eaters. They all spent lots of time working outdoors. Almost all of them used lots of pollen-rich honey in their diets. They all were either total vegetarians or ate only very little meat. They all were slim. They all were poor. And, they all were happy!

One man, 126 years old, told me:

"I've worked hard all of my life, but never had much money to worry about. I walk at least 5 miles every day, and ride a horse. I eat very little, and only when hungry—I never eat at regular times, but just when I feel really hungry. I was married four times, each time to a younger wife. Maybe this has helped me to stay young!" he finished with a chuckle.

The Russian Minister of Health told me a story of a Russian centenarian from Caucasus who lived to the respectable age of 146 years. When asked for the reasons for his enviable longevity, the man said:

"I've never had a boss over me. I have never been envious of what others have. And I have periodically rejuvenated myself by marrying three times!"

The above two cases seem to demonstrate that vibrant health, long life and sexual virility go hand in hand. Dr. Bernard Jensen, who has studied the lives of centenarians in Russia, Turkey, and Bulgaria, made a similar observation. Upon his return, he said:

"I've made a remarkable observation: almost all centenarians I've met have been married several times."

My conclusion is that we do not stop sexual activity because we grow old—we grow old because we stop sexual activity. Sexual interest and activity keep your adrenal and sex glands producing hormones, and these sex hormones will help to keep you young by stimulating and enhancing virtually all the vital functions in your body.

Recently, while making up an electoral list, Turkish authorities found the oldest man in Turkey, a 144-year-old farmer, Mustafa Tasci. He remarried at 83, when his first wife died, and he has 13 children and 50 grandchildren. Tasci is a vegetarian—he has never eaten meat in his life. He does not smoke, and has never drunk alcohol. He walks a mile and a half each day, and he still works in his orchard.

Mustafa Tasci's secret of long life is summed up in his words:

"Eat moderately; stay away from meat, smoke, and alcohol; work every day; and surround yourself with young children."

The oldest man I've met was Shirali Mislimov. He was 166 years of age at the time and lived in the Russian province of Azerbaidzhan, in the Caucasian mountains. Mislimov's formula for a long and happy life includes: clean air, natural foods, a slow pace, a kind heart, and a lot of work.

Here's his secret of long life in his own words, delivered in the poetic language of the Azerbaidzhan mountains:

"I was never in a hurry in my life, and I'm in no hurry to die now.

There are two sources of long life:

One is a gift of nature, and it is the pure air and clear water of the mountains, the fruit of the earth, peace, rest, and the soft warm climate of the highlands.

The second source is within us. He lives long who enjoys life and who bears no jealousy of others, whose heart harbors no malice or anger. who sings a lot and cries a little, who rises and retires with the sun, who likes to work, and who knows how to rest."

Regarding his diet, the 166-year-old Mislimov said: "I eat the usual food our people here have been eating for generations. Mostly fruits and homemade cheeses, and a very little meat. And I drink a little tea. I never eat when I am not hungry," he concluded.

One of the most inspiring examples of a long, happy, and useful life is the story of a Venetian nobleman of the 16th century, Luigi Cornaro.

A physical wreck, facing invalidism and death at the age of 36, rejected by contemporary doctors as incurable, he took his health into his own hands and began reading, studying, and experimenting in order to save his life. In a few years, he achieved robust and glowing health, and lived a happy and useful life in full possession of his physical and mental capacities, to the age of 103.

Luigi Cornaro wrote a book to tell others of his secrets of buoyant health and long life, originally titled,

A Sure and Certain Method for Attaining a Long and Healthy Life. The simplified title of the recent edition is, *The Art of Living Long.*

One of Cornaro's secrets is: "Not to satiate oneself with food is the science of health." He discovered that systematic undereating, or moderate eating, was the secret of feeling great. "My greatest discovery was that the less I ate, the better I felt," said Luigi Cornaro.

Carefully selecting his foods, he discovered that he felt best by eating grains, mostly in the form of bread, although he did use some animal foods in moderation.

He also discovered that diet alone was not sufficient to assure the highest level of health—that the influence of the mind and emotions had an important role to play in the overall health picture.

"I have also," he wrote, "preserved myself, as far as I have been able, from those other disorders from which it is more difficult to be exempt: I mean melancholy, hatred, and the other passions of the soul, which all appear greatly to affect the body."

In chapter 11, I told you about the renowned Chinese professor and herbalist, Li Chung Yun, who lived to be 256 years old. Researchers and writers who studied his life in detail, attributed his long life to his vegetarian diet and special rejuvenative herb teas which he drank all of his life: ginseng and gotu-kola.

Li Chung Yun himself, however, had a different idea for the reason for his long life. When asked to what he attributed his long life, he said:

"I attribute my long life to **INWARD CALM.**"

In all my studies of people who lived extraordinarily long lives in various parts of the world, I have found that in addition to all the other factors, such as sound nutrition of simple, unadulterated foods, scanty eating, poison-free environment, and plenty of exercise, they all possessed that unmistakable quality Professor Yun was talking about—**INWARD CALM**. They were contented, happy with their families, neighbors, and the other villagers. This sense of importance, of being useful, having the respect and adoration of families and neighbors is, in my opinion, an extremely important factor in longevity. Unfortunately, in the United States, oldsters usually face the opposite lot: they are excluded from a useful role in society, shoved into old peoples' homes, forgotten by families and relatives, feeling isolated, useless, and unloved.

Dr. Alexander Leaf, chief of medical services at Massachusetts General Hospital in Boston, made an extensive study in three sections of the world where people live extraordinarily long lives: The Andean village of Vilcabamba, Ecuador; the Hunza Kingdom in Kashmir; and the Black Sea coastal area of Abkhazia, in Russia.

In Abkhazia, Dr. Leaf met a 130-year-old woman who held the title of the fastest tea leaf picker on the collective farm where she worked.

In Hunza, he found a 110-year-old man who did a full day's work in the fields among younger men, binding hay on a steep hillside.

In Vilcabamba, he interviewed a 123-year-old man who had retired as a hunter 50 years ago, and was now actively engaged in farming.

All of these people were in excellent physical condition. Dr. Leaf's conclusion was that regular physical exercise, heredity, and a sense of importance, in addition to their generally low-calorie and low-protein diets, were important keys to a longer life.

I can still picture in my mind a 104-year-old man I met on one of my trips to Russia. He was living in a tiny mountainous village in Abkhazia and was herding sheep from horseback. At 104, he was still a superb horseman, able to mount his horse more easily than a typical American teenager could. When I asked him to what he attributed his long life, he said:

"I've had 3 wives, I have 17 children, 48 grandchildren, and many great and great-great-grandchildren. I am loved and respected by all of them, and I have much to live for. I have never had many possessions. I always worked for others, and I have never been jealous of what others have. I go to sleep with the sun, and get up with the sun. I eat simple things, and only when I am really hungry. I never smoked, and I taste a little wine on festive occasions. I love these mountains and the sheep and my horse, and I sing throughout most of the day. Life is wonderful when you can enjoy good health ..."

An American centenarian, Thomas Dayton, 107 years old, expressed his secret of long life thus:

"I kept my body active, but my mind at rest. People worry too much ... I've always taken care of myself physically, as well as mentally, by eating regular meals and getting plenty of sleep. I eat a lot of fruit—mostly apples, pears, and peaches. I drink goat's milk, because it has more nourishment than cow's milk. And I have never smoked."

Thomas Dayton married his second wife when he was 73.

I would like to conclude this chapter with the statement made by Alexander Leaf, M.D., who studied the lifestyles of centenarians to determine the causes of their exceptional longevity. Dr. Leaf says:

"I returned from my travels convinced that vigorous, active old age, free from debility and senility, is possible." (*Nutrition Today*, Vol. 8, Number 5, October/November, 1973.)

My own studies made in the same parts of the world that Dr. Leaf studied, as well as in other, less known or accessible areas, confirm Dr. Leaf's conclusion. The phenomenon of longevity seems to have many causes. But the most prominent contributing causes to long life seem to be:

1. Adequate nutrition provided by a simple diet of natural foods.
2. Systematic undereating.
3. Low-calorie, low-fat, low-protein, mostly vegetarian diet.
4. Plenty of exercise or outdoor work.
5. A certain genetic influence—centenarians usually had parents who likewise attained great age.
6. A stress-free, contented, happy, relaxed lifestyle, without worries, envy, hatred, or ambitions of wealth or power.
7. Feeling of being useful, loved, adored, and respected by their families and neighbors.
8. A positive, peaceful state of mind, or as 256-year-old Li Chung Yun put it, **Inward Calm.**

16

How Long Can You Live?

What is man's normal life span? You have just heard several centenarians, those who live to be 100 years of age and over, speak about their long lives. Can *you* live to be 100 or 120? Isn't the natural life span really only 70 years, or what the Bible refers to as threescore and ten?

In the Introduction, I mentioned the life-extension revolution that's going on in the United States right now. In the laboratories and universities, as well as in private longevity research centers, life-extension scientists are working feverishly to solve the mystery of aging and death. Some scientists regard physical death as an immutable law of nature, while others think that the human body is actually immortal, and death is unnatural. There are two basic theories regarding the natural life span, the mechanics of the aging processes, and death.

One theory is that our bodies are genetically and biologically programmed to die at a certain designated age. The studies of two researchers seem to support this theory. Leonard Hayflick and Paul Moorhead at the Wistar Institute in Philadelphia found that the human cell—previously thought to be able to divide indefinitely—can only divide a given number of times (this number known as the Hayflick Limit), then the cell division will slow down, and finally cease. Death ensues when cells can no longer divide or reproduce themselves. Hayflick discovered that human cells will divide and replicate approximately 50 times before they perish. Using Hayflick mathematics (50 cell divisions plus or minus 10), we can calculate that the potential human life span should be roughly 110 to 120 years.

Studies by Dr. W. Donner Denckla at Harvard University also support the theory of a genetically-programmed termination of life. According to his findings, the human pituitary gland secretes a "death hormone" which interferes with the body's ability to utilize thyroid hormone, thyroxine. Thyroxine directly controls the rate of cellular metabolism. Without thyroxine, cells cannot be properly fed; they stop reproducing, and eventually die.

The other theory, which seems to be more appealing to most researchers in the field of gerontology, is that the human machinery is constructed to function indefinitely provided the milieu and conditions are favorable and life-conducive. The reason we die is not because of a certain genetically programmed "aging clock," but because of multiple biological and biochemical derangements which interfere with the body's normal functions and cause premature death. Free-radicals, of which we spoke before, are cited as just one of the causes of premature aging and death. Amyloid (aging pigment) deposits, which impair cell function, are also cited as the cause of aging and death; so are deposits of another aging pigment, lipofuscin. Slowdown in endocrine hormone production and the body's diminished ability to use hormones as it ages are other manifestations of biochemical derangement that contribute to premature death.

My own thinking, based not only on my lifelong studies of the subject and on all the current scientific research data available in the field of gerontology and life-extension, but also on common sense, intuition, and insight, is that both above-mentioned theories are correct; that there aren't actually any contradictions between them.

One of the reasons for a seeming contradiction is the researchers' failure to comprehend the Biblical references to longevity which they, nevertheless, cite so frequently. Genesis 6:3 reads:

"And God said: My spirit shall not always dwell in man since he is of flesh; yet the number of his days shall be 120 years."

Then, in Psalms 90:10, it says:

"The days of our years are threescore and ten; and if by reason of strength, they be fourscore years, yet is their strength labor and sorrow; for it is cut off, and we fly away."

We have been conditioned to think that we are given a life span of threescore and ten by our Creator. This conditioning is responsible in a great part for a self-programmed biological "death clock" we have equipped ourselves with. And yet, this alleged divinely-designated life span of 70 years, in my view, is based on misunderstanding and misinterpretation of the Biblical texts. If you analyze the first quote from Genesis 6:3, you can see that, at the time of creation of man, God realized that, being "of flesh," man will not always follow the divine laws of life (if he did, he could live considerably longer, or even conceivably enjoy physical immortality), and, therefore, his life span *"shall be"* (emphasis mine) limited to 120 years. The second quote, from Psalms 90:10 is an historic chronicle of what actually happened. In poetic language, it decries the fact that the days of man's life now *are* threescore and ten; and even if someone "by reason of strength" can live ten years longer, he only has ten more years of "labor and sorrow" before he dies.

From these two Biblical quotes it seems clear to me that the human body was divinely designed and genetically and biologically programmed to function at optimal levels for 120 years. This is the span of life, the designated natural age of man. But, because of various violations of the laws of nature, dietary indiscretions, and other "sins and iniquities," man has gradually decreased his natural life span to threescore and ten (70 years).

This interpretation of the Biblical quotes agrees completely with the result of scientific research quoted earlier in this chapter. I believe that there is a genetically programmed "aging clock" present in the nucleus of every human cell. Thus, when the designated life span is reached (which for humans is 120 years), the special mechanism in the body control center, which is the combined body-mind-spirit life-energy center, activates the aging and life-terminating processes, which then bring the life-cycle to conclusion. Whether a "death hormone," as suggested by Dr. Denckla, is a part of this natural aging mechanism or not, is immaterial. What is important is to realize that our bodies *are* designed to function 120 years, or, in exceptional cases ("by the reason of strength") even longer, as many actual life cases in this book demonstrate so convincingly.

Those of us who do not live to be 120, do not die of old age—we kill ourselves prematurely by violating the basic laws of health and life. We overeat. We worry ourselves to death. We fail to get sufficient physical exercise. We fill our daily lives with negative emotions. We subject ourselves to physical and emotional stresses. We violate all the basic rules of optimal nutrition, eat too much protein and fat, eat processed, denatured junk foods. We smoke. We drink. We take toxic drugs. We subject ourselves to deadly chemicals in the air, water, and food. We are subjected to deadly radiation from

X-rays administered by doctors, chiropractors, and dentists. If anything, it is a miracle and a tribute to the extraordinarily durable human machinery, which we call the body, that we make it last even threescore and ten!

This brings us again to the basic tenet that I have stressed over and over in this book:

The ultimate secret of living long is to stay healthy and avoid diseases that age you prematurely and kill you before you reach your designated life span.

In other words, by avoiding factors that contribute to and accelerate the aging processes—by optimizing nutrition; by avoiding undue physical and emotional stresses; by getting sufficient exercise; by avoiding excess protein and fats in the diet; by avoiding X-rays and radiation; and by developing a positive, health-oriented, optimistic outlook on life—you can live your full divinely-designated span of life, enjoying youthful vitality and glowing health.

17

Are You
Shortening Your Life?

There are many ways of prolonging life, as we have seen so far. There are many secrets of looking and feeling young, secrets that "work," and secrets that don't. As one cynic said, "The best method of looking young is to lie about your age." There are quite a few famous health and long life experts who are doing just that. It always impresses the audiences when a speaker says, "Look at me, I am 82 years young!" How would they know that his birth certificate shows only 72?

By far the best method of prolonging life and looking and feeling young was expressed by Herbert Spencer, when he wrote:

"The whole secret of prolonging one's life consists in doing nothing to shorten it."

Dr. A. Ochsner, noted authority on aging, reported in the *Journal of American Geriatrics Society*, that premature senility can be controlled to a great extent by *avoiding factors that accelerate aging.*

As I said in the preceding chapter, if we would live in accordance with all the known laws of health, and *do nothing to cause disease and shorten life*, we would live to be at least 120 years of age, and enjoy youthful vitality, including sexual virility, throughout life. But man seems to go out of his way, using his ingenuity and inventiveness, to ruin his health and shorten his life. He is the only creature that spoils his food before he eats it—by frying, freezing, preserving, processing, and refining it. He poisons his air and water supply. Just imagine, he lets his water supply be poisoned with fluoride, a poison 15 times stronger than arsenic, which is now known to cause birth defects, kidney damage, heart injury, mongoloidism, and cancer! He depletes his soil by using chemicals that grow nutritionally inferior food which cannot sustain health. He ignores the basic law of life—need for motion—and shortens his life by a sedentary way of living, without sufficient physical exertion. Relaxation and peace of mind are imperative for health and long life, yet his life is filled with continuous mental and emotional stresses because he is haunted by the insatiable drive for more material wealth and power. He digs his own grave with his knife and fork, eating denatured, overprocessed, nutritionless, and poisoned foods which can only lead to serious and fatal diseases such as cancer, arthritis, heart disease, diabetes, etc.

Man, indeed, seems to do all he can to shorten his life!

Are you shortening *your* life?

I admit that we are all subjected to certain health-destroying factors that we cannot avoid. In this age of universal chemical pollution, it is not easy to live so that our health will not be endangered. Smog is difficult to escape. Equally difficult to escape are the thousands of health-destroying and life-shortening poisons in water and food. But a few things can be done to improve our individual lives and to protect our health to the greatest possible extent.

I must tell you a true story that happened recently—an example of how some people shorten their lives, largely by ignorance.

A couple in their middle years came to me for a

nutrition consultation. He was a balding, overweight man, looking to be around 60. She was the opposite: thin, appearing to be in her early fifties. I had my first surprise when I found that he was 46 and she was 39!

The couple told me that they were at the end of their rope; they were desperate for help. A reader of my books directed them to me. This is the kind of people a nutritionist usually sees. First they try everything else—medical specialists, expensive tests, fancy clinics, countless drugs, psychiatrists, more medical specialists—without receiving any help. Then they are ready, as a last-ditch attempt, to go to a nutritionist.

Here is their story, in his words:

"We had pretty good health until a few years ago. But then something happened. My wife became tired all the time, lost all of her interest in life—just laid in bed all day, complaining of aches and pains. Doctors couldn't find out what was wrong with her. They gave her hormone shots, suspecting hypothyroidism and premature menopause. But nothing helped. I began putting on weight a few years ago. I'm tired all the time, hardly able to drag my legs. I can't sleep. Our sex life is completely finished, too—I haven't touched my wife for a year. Not that she cares—she is so beat that sex is the farthest thing from her mind. I'm afraid of losing my job—I can't think straight, and I bark at everyone at work. I have a responsible executive position in my company and it's getting to be too much for me. After a few hours at the office, I'm ready to quit and go home. Coffee is the only thing that keeps me going. I drink a cup about every half hour."

As he talked, they both chain smoked. The interview revealed that this couple had been violating all of the known rules of health for decades. Both were heavy smokers and heavy drinkers. Their life was centered around nightly parties where they drank a lot of alcohol.

Their diet consisted largely of coffee—at least 10-15 cups a day—varied snacks, frozen dinners, sweets, and party snacks at night. They hardly ever ate fresh vegetables or fruits, nor whole grain bread or cereals. They drank no milk, but ate plenty of ice cream, and consumed lots of soft drinks. Their physical exercise was limited to walking from the bed to the bar, and walking to and from the car. They even used a push button to change the channels on the television. It is significant that *none of the doctors they visited had ever asked them what they ate or how they lived.*

When I suggested to them that their premature aging—her premature menopause, run-down condition, and gray hair; his obesity, lack of vitality, and sexual impotence—was brought about by their terrible living habits, their total disregard of all the elementary rules of health, they looked not only surprised, but also disappointed. They expected that I would give them a bottle of vitamin pills which would miraculously wipe out all their problems and restore their health and youth. Instead, I said that if they wanted their health and youth back, their libido and vitality restored, they must stop smoking, stop drinking alcohol, soft drinks, and coffee, and stop eating nutritionless junk foods. They must give up all-night parties and start regular physical exercise such as walking and jogging. They must begin eating health-building foods instead of health-destroying foods. In addition, I promised to outline for them a comprehensive revitalization and rejuvenation program with a special diet of health-building foods and special vitamins and food supplements.

It was difficult to convince them to make such a drastic change in their lifestyle. It had never occurred to them—and no doctor had ever suggested—that their conditions had anything to do with their way of living.

But, they had no choice: life was so miserable that they were willing to try anything.

Their program started with a short cleansing juice fast. Then a complete and rigid program of exercise, rest, and a diet of optimum nutrition—plenty of fresh vegetables and fruits, whole grain breads and cereals, seeds and nuts, yogurt, honey, pollen, brewer's yeast. No meat; no canned or processed foods; no white sugar or white bread; no sweets, ice cream, donuts, or soft drinks. They agreed to stop drinking alcohol completely, and to try to stop smoking.

It took three months for results to begin to show. I was amazed at their persistance. It took another three months before they could stop smoking. After six months, they reported to me that my program had "accomplished a miracle": they felt like new people! All tiredness was gone, her hair began to turn darker, menstrual irregularity disappeared, and she was full of vitality and slept like a baby. He lost over 30 pounds, he enjoyed his work at the office once more, and their sex life was completely straightened out. I've never seen a happier or more enthusiastic couple.

Are you shortening your life?

If you are, the true story I've just told you shows that you can make your life over, you can stop killing yourself and start growing younger! This book can show you the way. Turn back the pages and re-read Chapter 14. Follow the rejuvenative and health-building optimum diet I gave you, and avoid all the health-destroyers and life-shorteners I listed at the end of that chapter, as well as throughout the book. If you will do these things, I assure you that good things will begin to happen in your life: you will feel better; you will sleep better; you will lose those extra pounds you're carrying around; you will enjoy life more; you will ignore and overlook the inevitable daily irritations that used to drive you mad;

you will have a new surge of vitality, and if you have been losing interest in sex, you will experience new virility and libido that you have not known since your honeymoon!

How do I know that these things will happen to you? Simple: I have thousands of letters in my files from readers of my books and those for whom I have planned a personalized nutrition program—they all report miraculous changes in their lives after changing their living habits. This works by the simple natural law of cause and effect. You violate the basic laws of health, and you feel accordingly. You cannot fool Mother Nature. "Whatsoever ye sow, that also shall ye reap." Stop working *against nature* and start working *with nature.* Give nature a chance! Your body has a remarkable regenerative capacity. Remove all the health-destroyers and life-shorteners from your life—smoking, drinking, white sugar and white flour, processed, refined, denatured, and poisoned foods, drugs, and other chemicals— and follow the longevity diet described in Chapter 14. Make use of all the various health and longevity secrets from around the world which you have learned from this book, and *you will be amazed at the results!* You will begin to *grow younger* instead of growing older. Not only will most of your present health problems be solved, but you will feel and act like a new person. You will enjoy peace, contentment, happiness, and joy in living as you never have before.

Are you shortening your life and growing old prematurely?

You can change your life pattern and start growing younger—TODAY! Today is the beginning of the rest of your life. You may continue in the old rut, and grow older by the day—or you may change over and begin a new way of life which will help you to grow younger in body, mind, and spirit. It's up to you!

18

In a Nutshell

There are some book readers who are too impatient to read the whole book—they glance through the Table of Contents, the Introduction, and the last page to get the main points and to pick up some useful hints they can put into immediate practice. Some other readers of self-help books, by the time they come to the last chapter, tend to forget many important points they read about earlier in the book. For the benefit of these readers—and also in order to "put it all together" and present the whole stay-younger-longer program in a nutshell—I will now list all the do's and don'ts which, if conscientiously heeded and applied, will optimize your health and help give you a long and healthy life and youthful vitality.

Don'ts

- Don't smoke—anything!
- Don't abuse alcohol.
- Don't drink coffee or tea in excess; never use caffeine-containing soft drinks.

- Don't eat salt, sugar, or any processed, prepackaged, man-made foods.
- Don't use rancid or stale foods.
- Don't use any so-called "life-extending drugs": BHT and BNA, Centrophenoxine, BAPN, 2-MEA, L-Dopa, DMAE, Thiodipropionate, Penicillamine, Sulfadiazine, to mention a few. These drugs are hailed by some "longevists" as effective life-extenders, but there is no reliable scientific research that proves their effectiveness or safety.
- Don't subject yourself to X-rays, unless it is absolutely necessary (90% of all X-rays taken today are unnecessary).
- Don't overeat. Systematic undereating is one of the most solidly proven life-extending factors.
- Don't eat meat; or reduce its consumption to an absolute minimum.
- Don't eat a heavy breakfast early in the morning; make lunch your largest meal.
- Don't drink chlorinated and/or fluoridated water.
- Don't overextend yourself; rest and relaxation are vital for your health and long life.

Do's

- Eat a low-protein, low-fat, high-natural-carbohydrate diet of high-quality natural foods, as outlined in this book. This is a *must* for vigorous health and long life.
- Supplement your diet with special vitamins, minerals, trace elements and other food supplements and specific foods which have been proven to have age-retarding and life-extending properties.
- Use regularly specific rejuvenative and age-retarding herbs that are mentioned in this book.
- Eat only when really hungry.

- Get plenty of exercise or outdoor work. Remember my oft-quoted statement: "It is better to eat junk foods and exercise a lot than to eat health foods and not exercise at all."
- Drink pure, naturally hard (mineralized) water from wells or springs.
- Get plenty of pure air and sunshine—these are essential for your health.
- Go on a periodic juice fast. Fasting is the royal road to optimum health and long life.
- Develop a positive, peaceful, loving, and forgiving state of mind. A happy disposition, hope, and faith are the most important ingredients for optimum health and a long, happy, fulfilling, and joyous life.

Conclusion

Why Live Long?

It is hardly worth-while to learn how to live long if you have to live a life of suffering from one agonizing disease after another. A long life makes sense only if it can be lived in vibrant health and enjoyed in the active, productive pursuit of one's most treasured interests.

Unfortunately, there are very few people around who are really enjoying perfect health. Most are sick, semi-sick, or half-healthy. Really healthy persons have become so rare that the standards of good health are no longer very high. One man, whom I tried to admonish to stop smoking, said to me, "Why should I? I am perfectly healthy. Smoking hasn't hurt my health!" Yet, he consumes a handful of pills each day—aspirins for his headaches, alkalizers for his indigestion, laxatives, tranquilizers, and sleeping aids. He was in the hospital twice during the last year, he has high blood pressure, and wears dentures at the age of 38. "Perfectly healthy," indeed!

Many feel that if they are still standing on their feet and are not confined to a hospital bed, they are in "good health." But a study conducted by Tulane University in Louisiana, showed that 92% of all Americans—92 out of every 100!—have something wrong with them and are suffering from some form of physical or mental disorders!

No wonder I so often hear the following comment, especially when I lecture to groups not previously exposed to health-building ideas:

"Why should I stop enjoying such fruits of civilization as alcohol, tobacco, and gourmet foods I like—only to be assured of a few more years of life? I'd rather enjoy eating, drinking, and doing what I like, and die a few years earlier!"

First, if eating, drinking, smoking, and doing "what you like" would not affect your health detrimentally, but would allow you to function at the optimal level of health until the time you die, you would have a point there. But when drinking, smoking, overeating and other "enjoyable" abuses destroy your health and age you prematurely, then they defeat their purpose, because you can hardly *enjoy* living when you are sick and half-dead.

Second, the reason for changing your eating and living habits is not just to live a few more years, but *to live whatever years you are going to live in buoyant health—and ENJOYING THEM—in youthful vitality and vigor.*

Moreover, the real purpose of attaining better physical health and a longer life is not just the mere enjoyment of life, but a higher, divine purpose for which life was given to us. All endeavors toward attaining better health and extended longevity would be a wasted effort unless the healthy body is used as a worthy temple for the spirit to dwell in and develop. I believe that the true purpose of our lives is not just living a long time, or the building of magnificent bodies, developing bulging biceps and lovely complexions, but perfecting and refining our divine spirits, and becoming more God-like. "Be ye perfect, even as your Father, which is in heaven, is perfect," said the Man from Nazareth. Our life on this planet, at this time in history, is just a short episode in the eternal divine plan of human development—a schooling period aimed at improving and perfecting our human and divine characteristics. Only those who are unaware of the high goal and divine purpose of human life talk about "eat, drink, and be merry."

Although most of the pages in this book are devoted to the discussion of the physical and biological aspects of achieving optimum health and long life, I would not wish to leave my readers with the impression that I consider the mere attainment of a long life, or even a high level of physical health, to be the sole purpose and goal in life. As worthwhile and enjoyable as good health can be, it won't guarantee happiness and fulfillment. We have all seen people who are in perfect physical health, yet unhappy and miserable. On the other hand, I have known those who were afflicted with obvious misfortunes and ill health—yes, even dying of a terminal illness—yet they have overlooked or ignored their seeming burdens, and, instead of falling into the trap of self-pity, have radiated joy and happiness, and shown love and concern for the welfare and happiness of others.

True and lasting happiness comes from the realization of the divine origin and purpose of all life, and from the directing of our own lives and channeling of all our energies toward the expression and exemplification of the divine plan in our daily lives. Man is an immortal spiritual being. He has always lived, and upon leaving this earthly plane, will continue his eternal progression. This short episode of earthly existence is nothing but a learning process; specifically, an intensive course designed to teach love—love for our fellow men, and love for God. Upon graduation, we return to God to continue on our eternal path of progression toward spiritual perfection and becoming more God-like. Improving one's health, building a strong, disease-free body, and living a long life on this earth can be rewarding and joyous experiences, but only if we understand the divine plan for our lives, keep priorities right, and show our love of God by giving and sharing our love and happiness with others. We receive only in the measure in which we are able and willing to give. By becoming more loving, more compassionate, more forgiving and more sharing, we not only will improve the health of our bodies and extend the enjoyable and happy years of this life, but we will also be refining and perfecting our spirits that will live forever.

INDEX

Sexual vigor, 77, 107, 124, 127, 136, 172
Sherman, Dr. Henry G., 139
Skin
  aging of, 20, 23, 28, 36
  discolorations of, 124
  disorders, 79, 106
  dryness of, 72, 126
  wrinkled, 122, 128
  youthful appearance of, 128
Smoking, 151, 172, 176, 181, 189, 192
Spiritual attitude, importance of, 11, 120, 193-194
Spiritual awareness, 55, 170
Sprouting, 135, 192
Stone, Dr. I., 20
Stress, 12, 110, 123, 135, 139, 163
Sugar, 152, 187, 190
Sunflower seeds, 59, 68, 129, 135, 142
Sunshine, 169, 191

T

Tappel, Dr. Aloys L., 121, 124
Testosterone, 14, 107
Thyroxine, 179
Trace elements, 77
Tsitsin, Nicolai, 61

U

Ulcers, 63, 124
Unsaturated fatty acids, 99, 132, 142
Uric acid, 13, 54, 104

V

Varicose veins, 124
Vegetable oils, 146, 152
Vegetable proteins, 88, 142-143
Vegetarian diet, 76, 85, 89, 91, 112, 140, 171, 172, 174, 177
Virility, 21, 58, 84, 99, 107, 183
  lecithin and, 131
  longevity and, 172
  minerals and, 134, 136
  vitamins and, 21, 121, 124, 129
Virtanen, Dr. A.I., 65
Visualization, 166
Vitamins, anti-aging
  A, 125-126
  B_1, 127

B_2, 128
B_3, 128
B_5, 127, 130
B_6, 129
B_{12}, 62, 77
B_{15}, 128
C, 16, 19, 21, 24, 124-125
choline, 132
D, 132
E, 121-124
folic acid, 129-130
inositol, 132
K, 132
PABA, 129, 130
Voronoff, Dr. Serge, 9

W

Waerland, Are, 55, 116
Water, 16, 48-49, 169
  diabetes and, 16
  distilled, 50, 94, 149
  fluoridated, 184, 190
  hard, 149, 191
  heart disease and, 149
  minerals in, 16, 49, 92-94, 136, 149
  osteoporosis and, 16, 93
  soft, 93
  with meals, 157
Wheat germ, 135, 152
Whey, 25-29
Williams, Dr. Roger, 20, 127
Work, as longevity factor, 171-172
Wrinkles, 20, 72, 122, 124, 151

X

X-rays, 182, 190

Y

Yogurt, homemade, 45, 57
Youth doctors, 8, 9, 11, 169
Youth drugs, 8, 72, 138
Youth vitamin, 112

Z

Zabel, Dr. Werner, 30, 52, 55
Zinc, 68, 78, 130, 134-135

ABOUT THE AUTHOR

Paavo Airola, Ph.D., N.D., is an inter-nationally-recognized nutritionist, naturo-pathic physician, educator, and award-winning author. Raised and educated in Europe, he studied biochemistry, nutrition, and natural healing in biological medical centers of Sweden, Germany, and Switzer-land. He lectures extensively world-wide, both to professionals and laymen, holding yearly educational seminars for physicians. He has been a visiting lecturer at many universities and medical schools, including the Stanford University Medical School.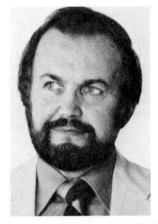

Dr. Paavo Airola is the author of fourteen widely-read books, notably his two inter-national best-sellers, *How to Get Well*, and *Are You Confused? How to Get Well* is the most authoritative and practical manual on natural healing in print. It is used as a textbook in several universities and medical schools, and regarded as a reliable reference manual, the "Bible of Natural Healing," by doctors, researchers, nutritionists, and students of health and holistic healing. Dr. Airola's book, *Hypoglycemia: A Better Approach*, has revolution-ized the therapeutic concept of this insidious, complex, and devastating affliction. The American Academy of Public Affairs issued Dr. Airola the Award of Merit for his book on arthritis.

Dr. Airola's monumental work, *Everywoman's Book*, is a great new contribution in the field of holistic medicine. It not only confirms Dr. Airola's unchallenged leadership in the field of nutrition and holistic healing, but demonstrates his genius as an original thinker, philosopher, and profound humanitarian.

The Airola Diet & Cookbook is Dr. Airola's newest book. It contains not only 300 delicious and nutritious recipes and Dr. Airola's Weight Loss Program, but also the most thorough presentation to date of the scientific basis for the Airola Optimum Diet — the world-famous diet of supernutrition for superhealth.

Dr. Airola is President of the International Academy of Biological Medicine; a member of the International Naturopathic Association; and a member of the International Society for Research on Civilization Diseases and Environment, the prestigious Forum for world-wide research founded by Dr. Albert Schweitzer. Dr. Airola is listed in the *Directory of International Biography, The Blue Book, The Men of Achievement, Who's Who in American Art, Who's Who in the West,* and *Canadian Who's Who.*

DR. PAAVO AIROLA'S WORK

"EVERYWOMAN'S BOOK is a massive accomplishment by a single author. Comprehensively documented. Invaluable qualities of judgement, assessment, evaluation, and selectivity, and the analytical deliberation, ethical standards, and mature wisdom distinguish Dr. Airola as a giant in the field. His book deserves to be immediately read and then used as a reference by families throughout our country. We will recognize true progress in creating a healthy American population when Benjamin Spock's influence of decades ago is replaced by Paavo Airola and his new book."

Dr. Robert S. Mendelsohn, M.D.; author; Associate Professor,
University of Illinois, College of Medicine; President,
National Health Federation; Chicago, IL

"HOW TO GET WELL is extremely practical and helpful for the reader, and a giant example of research and work. I will refer to it many times, giving you credit all the way . . . Many thanks, and congratulations!"

Linda Clark, M.A., author, nutritionist, Carmel, CA

"I am congratulating you for your pioneering work. It will contribute to the freedom of thought and therapeutic alternatives — and, thus, to the improvement of the health standards in the world."

Dr. L.E. Essén, M.D., Sweden

"May I thank you for your exemplar teachings in the field of Biological Medicine from which I have derived a lot of benefits as one of your many students. I frequently refer to your excellent books for helpful answers to vexing problems of my patients and friends"

Dr. Stanley F. Hansen, M.D., F.A.P.A., El Cajon, CA

"I have read all of your books and regard you as the ultimate authority on health matters. HOW TO GET WELL is my nutrition Bible."

M.H., Lantana, FL

"Dr. Airola's HOW TO GET WELL Is undoubtedly the book of the century! He is America's foremost nutritionist and is in the unique position of having his ideas received favorably by a growing number of medical doctors."

Scott Smith, Assoc. Editor, Vegetarian Times

"Your book (EVERYWOMAN'S BOOK) is a masterpiece! It should be read by every woman —preferably together with her husband!"

Dr. Abram Ber, M.D., Phoenix, AZ

"EVERYWOMAN'S BOOK answers every question any woman could ever have. My only regret is that it wasn't published sooner — many women would have been saved a lot of unnecessary suffering. Your book will be a reference for me for the rest of my life."

Rebecca Clarkes, Editor, ALIVE Magazine, Canada

"I have just read your book on cancer. It is such a beautiful work, honest, concise, and well documented. You are doing such a good work in reawakening mankind's consciousness to natural healing resources within us which can enable us to reach new heights in health and awareness."

Dr. Jeff Migdow, M.D., Summit Station, PA

"Thank you for your wonderful books. You are spreading an important message all over the world which shows suffering mankind the way to better health and happiness."

Ebba Waerland, Author, healer. Switzerland

"EVERYWOMAN'S BOOK is fantastic. I cannot relive my life but I can sure live the rest of it better and teach my children with the help of your books."

Mrs. S.K., Toronto, Canada

"I am using Dr. Airola's books as textbooks in my Honors Class on nutrition-health relationship. I know of no better author on such matters."

Dr. Louis Junker, Ph.D., Prof., Western Michigan University

"Never have I read such a fascinating, exciting, and complete health manual. EVERYWOMAN'S BOOK is the most needed book of the century! In my own practice I rely heavily on the information and proven practices advocated in Dr. Airola's books."

Dr. Mary Ann Kibler, M.D., Corry, PA

"My mother-in-law was supposed to have died of cancer two years ago. After following instructions in your book, doctors cannot find a trace of cancer in her."

S.Z., Hillsboro, CA

"HOW TO GET WELL is wonderful. No one deserves more than yourself the success you are having."

Betty Lee Morales, nutritionist; President, Cancer Control Society, Los Angeles, CA

"Without doubt, HOW TO GET WELL is the best and the most informative book on natural healing ever published. Finally we have a book that we can recommend to every one of our customers —and feel good about it."

M.H., health food store owner, Charleston, WV

"The best and most effective treatment for low blood sugar was developed by Dr. Paavo Airola and outlined in his book, HYPOGLYCEMIA: A BETTER APPROACH. Up to 80% of my patients have low blood sugar and I treat them with the Airola diet with excellent results — it is far superior to the traditional high protein diet."

Dr. Willem H. Khoe, M.D., President, Acupuncture Research Institute, Las Vegas, NV

"For years I have been impressed by your rational, independent thinking, your comprehensive approach to health and nutrition questions, and your flexible, adaptable orientation to new information and new ideas. I personally have derived great benefit from your books and am always recommending them to others."

J.D. Shapiro, Assoc. Prof., Memorial University of Newfoundland, Canada

"Your book, ARE YOU CONFUSED?, is the most important health book ever published."

Dr. R. Huckabay, N.D., D.C., Los Angeles, CA

"I feel that your fasting book is a masterpiece. I have fasted many times in the past on water, but your juice fasting method is superior. I am on my 28th day of a juice fast, and feel great!

F.C.W., Phoenix, AZ

"After having suffered for three years with severe symptoms of hypoglycemia, such as periodic loss of coordination, dizziness, and exhaustion, I found your book, HYPOGLYCEMIA: A BETTER APPROACH — and bless the day I did! Now, one month later, no more symptoms — I feel great!"

S.M., La Jolla, CA

"EVERYWOMAN'S BOOK is a book every woman should own and treasure. I certainly will! It is a remarkable achievement and certainly your best book to date."

Dr. Susan Smith Jones, Ph.D., Los Angeles, CA

"No doubt in my mind about it: you are the Number One nutritionist and the most knowledgeable health writer."

A.S., Reg. Therapist, Escondido, CA

"I am an M.D. with an open mind. I am employing your programs, described in THERE *IS* A CURE FOR ARTHRITIS and they are actually doing wonders for my patients."

Dr. T.J., M.D., Grafton, WV

"I have read widely on nutrition, but your books are, in my opinion, the most balanced in emphasis and sound in conclusions of any that I have read. I give your books to my patients and they are most appreciative of them."

Dr. J.S.J., M.D., Carmel, CA

"EVERYWOMAN'S BOOK is the best to-date by a Holistic author placing an emphasis on the integration of the Body, Mind, and Spirit."

Dr. J.H. Coyle, M.D., D.Psych., Scottsdale, AZ

"I became a follower of your approach to health a few years ago when I discovered ARE YOU CONFUSED?. I found your attitude, your sense of responsibility to the public, and your method of formulating principles very refreshing, and rare. I will always be grateful that I read EVERYWOMAN'S BOOK before starting a family. I can't say enough good about it — it is a timely and altogether wonderful book. I am glad, too, that you, who hold such a recognized position in the health field, emphasize so strongly the spiritual and moral aspects of health. This is what America needs now. Thank you for your concern for people."

J.L.S., Gig Harbor, WA

"Your book, HOW TO GET WELL, is sensational! I am impressed with the way you conceived and constructed it, with your fabulous and expert presentation of the philosophy of Biological Medicine and with the common and academic sense it makes . . . you rendered a great service to a disease-ridden mankind."

Dr. H. Rudolph Alsleben, M.D., Anaheim, CA

"I have been using your ideas in my practice for several years now with excellent results. There are people back on the job after being told by their prior physicians to retire because of disability with their arthritis. Keep up the good work."

Dr. Harvey Walker, Jr., M.D., Ph.D., Clayton, MO

"We respect you for the fact that you are not out to just make money from the public by lending your name to breads, soups, teas, herbs, vitamins, etc., etc., as so many nutritionists do, but that you are sincerely interested in better health for all people. We have all of your books and frequently loan them to friends to get them started on the Airola Diet."

R.J.M., Huntington Beach, CA

"My congratulations and heartfelt thanks on behalf of suffering humanity . . . Only through such research and writings as yours that the tide is ever going to turn from passive disease thinking to positive health thinking."

Dr. T.F., N.D., Pasadena, CA

"God bless you in your wonderful work."

Carlson Wade, renowned author, NY, NY

"Your service to mankind cannot be overestimated. You are a leader in the natural health field and your books are invaluable both for laymen and professionals. Keep up the good work!"

Dr. W.D. Currier, M.D., Pasadena, CA

"I have read through HOW TO GET WELL many times and have received both practical and philosophical information of great help to me."

Dr. L.M. Lawrence, D.M.D., Wharton, NJ

"I have been using and profitting from your books for several years. Thank you for the help and joy your books have added to the life of this one person. But even more, thank you for the information and help you so tirelessly make available to the whole human family."

Mrs. E.L., Scottsdale, AZ

"Thank you for HOW TO GET WELL. I refer to it daily for my family and clients."

Dr. Joy H. Bailey, Ed.D., George State University

"Your book, ARE YOU CONFUSED? is a masterpiece. It should be must reading for everyone who wants to achieve better health."

Robert Yaller, author, Venice, CA

"EVERYWOMAN'S BOOK is truly a treasure chest! Each chapter is a jewel and an obvious product of thorough research."

Dr. Virginia Flanagan, M.D., Assistant Clinical Professor, U.C.L.A.; Director, International College of Applied Nutrition; Sherman Oaks, CA

"If EVERYWOMAN'S BOOK was used as a major text in the curriculum of our medical schools, we would have a healthier and stronger America."

Dr. J.P. Hutchins, M.D., Fallbrook CA

"Thank God for such eye-opening knowledge about nutrition. Information in your books saved my life. A billion thanks!"

S.W., Los Angeles, CA

"You have absolutely no idea how much your book, HYPOGLYCEMIA: A BETTER APPROACH, has meant to me; it is literally a life-saver!"

G.W.K., Redding, CA

"In our clinic I have noticed a great improvement ever since we started using Dr. Airola's concepts. Before I was one of the 'Pasteurian thinkers', but Dr. Airola changed that. My sincerest thanks and compliments!"

Dr. R.T. Kennedy, Ph.D., N.D., St. Thomas, Ontario

"I wish to compliment you on your brilliant and dynamic presentations of contemporary health problems and how they can be overcome in a most logical and convincing sequence. I have received great pleasure and stimulation from reading your books and feel you have given to the people of the Western world some priceless teachings which they are so pathetically in need of."

Dr. M.O. Garten, N.D., author, naturopathic physician,
San Jose, CA

"Dr. Airola is not only the most knowledgeable but also the most honest writer of them all."

Dr. Kathleen M. Power, D.C., Pasadena, CA

"Congratulations on a truly excellent and much needed book. I literally could not put it down. The material in EVERYWOMAN'S BOOK is comprehensive, well-organized, and presented with clarity."

Dr. Michael E. Rosenbaum, M.D.; Vice President, Orthomolecular
Medical Society; Mill Valley, CA

"I cannot tell you in words what your wonderful book, HOW TO GET WELL, has meant to me. For ordinary people like me who are earnestly seeking information leading to better health — and there must be thousands of us — this book is a God-send answer. May the Lord bless you for this wonderful work of yours!"

I.L., Honolulu, HI

"I have read many books on nutrition but none of them have explained in such clear, concise, easy to understand terms the relationship of diet to our emotional, physical and spiritual wellbeing."

L.R., Hyattsville, MD

"Next to my Bible, HOW TO GET WELL is the best book I have ever read!"

Mrs. K.B., Dayton, OH

"Your HOW TO GET WELL book is tremendous. How I wish it had crossed my path years ago."

E.W.M., Chula Vista, CA

"Thank you for your wonderful book, HOW TO GET WELL. I had acne for 12 years. I've tried everything. Nothing really helped. So when I read your treatment for acne, I didn't have much faith in it, but decided to try it anyway. Imagine my surprise when my acne cleared up 90%!!! As long as I stay on your program my face remains clear — for the first time in years!"

J.A., Carlsbad, CA

"I have read all of your books and consider you to be the most important figure in the alternative health field."

C.M. Bryant, E.B., P.H.E.; Director, Natural Health
Institute; Glendale, CA

"EVERYWOMAN'S BOOK is magnificent: It is one of your most important works. Your conclusions are well-documented by massive scientific references. I commend you for it."

Dr. Michael L. Gerber, M.D., Mill Valley, CA

"Thank you for the priceless gift of your hardwon knowledge and your generous spirit which seeks to aid and guide the sick onto alternate and safer paths to healing of body and mind."

Mrs. C.D.T., Hatboro, PA

(There are hundreds of similar unsolicited comments in publishers' files.)

BHA/BHT   P.11-12   <u>NO</u>

P.14 Endocrine Glands (the Secret?)

Roses P.19-20 = <u>VITC</u> on Adrenal Glands P.21
(Hips)

P.22 Sex hormones #1 Aging Begins = <u>VIT.C</u>
P.22 Cells oxyggenation
P.77 Iodine in Sea Weed
    P.78 Thyroid = Sex Drive/libido
         Regulates Cell Oxygen

<u>Best Foods</u>   P.62 Honey
        P.64 Bee Pollen.

Buckwheat   P.25 Whey +
         (Sour Milks)
        P.28-29 (Butter + Chees

        P.39 millet (Buckwheat)
          proteins

        P.40 Sour Dough Rye Brea
         L Recipe

        P.44 Cultured
         45 Recipes

        P.76 Seaweed